SUREWAY FOR WEIGHT LOSS

An effective beginners guide on how to lose weight permanently

(for both children, adults and pregnant mothers)

i

Contents

INTRODUCTION

Obesity is a medical disorder in which a person's weight or body fat levels are too high to be healthy. It is a complicated condition characterized by an excess of body fat. Obesity is more than a cosmetic problem. It is a medical condition that can lead to severe illnesses such as type 2 diabetes, hypertension, and asthma. Obesity increases the risk of stroke, cancer, heart disease, liver disease, and kidney disease. Obesity has been linked to depression and low self-esteem in people.

There are indeed a host of reasons that certain people struggle to stop being obese. Obesity is usually caused by a combination of genetic and environmental factors, as well as personal diet and workout choices.

The good news is that even small weight loss can help or avoid obesity-related health issues. Weight loss can be achieved by dietary changes, increased physical activity, and behavioral changes. Obesity can also be treated with prescription drugs and weight-loss techniques.

If a person's body mass index is high, a doctor may often conclude that they are obese. The BMI is a body fat calculation dependent on a person's weight in relation to his or her height and age. Any individual with a BMI of 25-29.9 is deemed overweight whereas a BMI of 30 or higher is considered obese

If your body mass index (BMI) is 30 or higher, you are considered obese. To calculate your BMI, multiply your weight in pounds by your height in inches squared, then multiply by 703. Alternatively, multiply your weight in kilograms by your squared height in meters.

BMI = kg/m2, where kg represents a person's in kg and m2 represents their height in meters squared.

BMI	Weight status
18.5 and below	Underweight
18.5-24.9	Normal
25.0-29.9	Overweight
30.0 and above	Obesity

BMI offers a fair measure of body fat for the majority of people. However, since BMI does not specifically quantify body fat, some individuals, such as muscular athletes, may have a BMI that falls into the obesity category while having no excess body fat.

Other factors that influence a person's weight and body shape include the waist-to-hip ratio (WHR), waist-to-height ratio (WTHR), and the volume and distribution of fat on the body.

Obesity and excess weight can raise a person's risk of developing a variety of health problems, including metabolic syndrome, arthritis, and some forms of cancer.

Hypertension, type 2 diabetes, and cardiovascular disease are among the symptoms of metabolic syndrome.

Obesity may be prevented or reduced by maintaining a healthy weight or losing weight by diet and exercise. Surgery may be needed in some cases.

Ask your doctor about obesity treatment if you're worried about weight-related health issues. You and your doctor will explore your weight-loss choices and assess your health risks.

Causes of Obesity

Obesity occurs when you consume more calories than you burn through exercise and normal daily routines, despite genetic, behavioral, metabolic, and hormonal factors. Continue reading to learn why obesity occurs. The possible causes include;

Consumption of Excessive Calories

If a person's diet consists primarily of fruits, vegetables, and whole grains, they are less likely to become obese.

When a person consumes more calories than their body uses for energy, the excess calories are stored as fat. Obesity and excess weight will occur as a result of this.

Furthermore, certain foods, especially those high in fats and sugars, are more likely to cause weight gain.

The following foods have been proven to increase the risk of weight gain:

Fast foods

- Fried foods, like French fries
- Meats that are fatty and refined
- Several dairy products
- Pastries, ready-made breakfast cereals, and cookies all contain added sugar.
- Foods including ketchup and many other canned and processed foods contain secret sugars.
- Juices with added sugar, sodas, and alcoholic beverages
- Packaged, high-carb foods, like bread and bagels
- High-fructose corn syrup used as a sweetener in some processed foods, including savory things like ketchup.

Excessive consumption of these foods combined with inadequate exercise can contribute to weight gain and obesity.

Even if a person eats a diet high in fruits, vegetables, whole grains, and water, they are still at risk of gaining weight if they overeat or if genetic factors, such as obesity, increase their risk.

They are, however, more advised to eat a diverse diet and maintain a healthy weight. Fresh fruits and vegetables, as well as whole grains, contain fiber, which keeps you fuller for longer and promotes good digestion.

1.   Living A Sedentary Lifestyle

Obesity can be avoided with regular physical activity. Most people nowadays are much more inactive than their parents and grandparents were.

Sedentary behaviors include the following:

- Working in an office rather than doing factory work
- Instead of engaging in physical activity outdoors, people prefer to play video games on their computers.
- Driving most of the time Instead of walking or cycling

An individual burn less calories if they do not move around much.

Physical activity also influences how a person's hormones work, and hormones influence how the body absorbs food.

Physical activity has been shown in a number of studies to help keep insulin levels stable, and that unstable insulin levels can contribute to weight gain.

Lifestyle including routine (including physical activity) has been described as a key factor for sustaining and improving many aspects of health, including insulin sensitivity. Physical exercise does not have to be done in a gym. Physical labor, such as walking or riding, stair climbing, and domestic chores, all help.

The nature and intensity of exercise, on the other hand, will have an impact on how much it affects the body in the short and long term.

2.   Insufficient Sleep

Sleep deprivation has been linked to an increased risk of gaining weight and developing obesity, according to research.

From 1977 to 2012, researchers analyzed data on over 28,000 children and 15,000 adults in the United Kingdom. They concluded in 2012 that sleep deprivation increased the risk of obesity in both adults and children. Children as young as 5 years old were affected by the changes.

Sleep deprivation, according to the researchers, can contribute to obesity by causing hormonal changes that increase appetite. When a person does not get enough sleep, their body produces ghrelin, an appetite-stimulating hormone. At same time, sleep deprivation causes a decrease in the development of leptin, an appetite suppressant hormone.

Consumption of liquid fructose

A study published in the World Journal of Gastroenterology by a team from the University of Barcelona sheds light on how liquid fructose, a form of sugar found in beverages, can alter lipid energy metabolism and lead to fatty liver and metabolic syndrome.

Metabolic syndrome is characterized by diabetes, cardiovascular disease, and high blood pressure. Metabolic syndrome is more likely to occur in obese people. The scientists noticed a difference in the rats' metabolism after feeding them a 10% fructose solution for 14 days.

Scientists agree that high fructose intake is linked to obesity and metabolic syndrome. The use of high-fructose corn syrup to sweeten beverages and other foods has sparked concerns among authorities.

Obesity caused by fructose intake is associated with a high risk of type 2 diabetes, according to animal studies. Researchers published the findings of experiments involving young rats in 2018. After drinking fructose syrup, they too experienced metabolic changes, oxidative stress, and inflammation.

"Increased fructose intake may be an effective predictor of metabolic risk in young people," the researchers write.

To avoid these concerns, they argue for changes in young people's diets.

High-fructose corn syrup should be avoided. High-fructose corn syrup, which has been related to an increased risk of obesity, is widely used in ready-made sauces.

High-fructose corn syrup is present in the following foods:

- Sodas, energy drinks, and sports drinks are all examples of carbonated beverages.
- Ice cream and candy
- creamer for coffee
- Sauces and condiments, which include salad dressings, ketchup, and barbecue sauce
- Yogurt, juices, and canned foods are examples of sweetened foods.
- Bread and other ready-made snack foods
- Cereal bars

Reduce the consumption of corn syrup and other additives by doing the following:

- ✓ Before you buy, read the labels.

- ✓ If at all possible, choose unsweetened or minimally processed foods.
- ✓ Make your own salad dressings and other baked goods at home.
- ✓ Other sweeteners can be used in certain foods, but they can have negative impacts as well.

3.   Medications and weight gain

Weight gain is a side effect of certain drugs. Some medications caused people to gain weight over a span of months, according to the results of a study and meta-analysis published in The Journal of Clinical Endocrinology and Metabolism in 2015.

Olanzapine, quetiapine, and risperidone are examples of atypical antipsychotics.

Gabapentin and other anticonvulsants and mood stabilizers

Tolbutamide and other hypoglycemic drugs

Rheumatoid arthritis is treated with glucocorticoids.

Some antidepressants

Some drugs, on the other hand, can cause weight loss. If you're beginning a new medication and are worried about your weight, ask your doctor if the drug is likely to affect your weight.

4. Family inheritance and impacts

The amount of body fat you store and where that fat is distributed will be influenced by the genes you inherit from your parents. Genetics can also influence how efficiently your body turns food into energy, how your appetite is regulated, and how calories are burned during exercise.

Obesity is a trait that runs in families. That isn't all due to the fact that they have the same genes. Family members have a propensity to eat and exercise in similar ways.

5.   Social and economic issues

Obesity is attributed to social and economic causes. Obesity is impossible to stop if there are no safe places to walk or exercise. Similarly, you may not have been taught safe cooking techniques or have limited access to nutritious foods. Furthermore, the people you spend time with may have an effect on your weight — you're more likely to develop obesity if you have obese friends or family.

6.   Age

Obesity can strike anyone at any age, including children. Hormonal changes and a less healthy lifestyle, however, raise the risk of obesity as you get older. Furthermore, as you grow older, the body's muscle mass decreases. Lower muscle mass is associated with a slower metabolism. These modifications often decrease calorie requirements, making it more difficult to lose weight. You'll gain weight if you don't actively control what you eat and become more physically active as you grow older.

Other Factors

Pregnancy: During pregnancy, it is normal to gain weight. After the baby is born, some women find it difficult to lose this weight. Obesity in women can be increased as a result of this weight gain. Breast-feeding can be the most effective way to lose pregnancy weight.

Quitting smoking: Weight gain is often related to smoking cessation. And for others, it can result in enough weight gain to be considered obese. This also occurs as people turn to food to help them cope with the effects of quitting smoking. However, stopping smoking is also a safer choice for your wellbeing in the long term than continuing to smoke. Your doctor will assist you in avoiding weight gain after you stopped smoking.

Stress: Obesity can be triggered by a number of external factors that influence your mood and wellbeing. When people are nervous, they tend to crave more high-calorie foods.

Microbiome: What you eat has an effect on your gut bacteria, which can lead to weight gain or trouble losing weight.

Past efforts to lose weight: Previous attempts at weight loss that were accompanied by a rapid weight gain could lead to more weight regain. This phenomenon, also known as yo-yo dieting, can cause your metabolism to slow down.

Having one or more of these risk factors does not imply that you are doomed to become obese. Remember that diet, physical activity and exercise, and behavioral improvements can also help to minimize risk factors.

Complications of Obesity
Obese people are more likely to experience a variety of potentially serious health issues, such as:

Heart disease and strokes: Obesity increases the risk of high blood pressure and elevated cholesterol levels, all of which are risk factors for heart disease and stroke.

Type 2 diabetes: Obesity will influence how the body regulates blood sugar levels by changing how insulin is used. Insulin resistance and diabetes are more likely as a result of this.

Certain cancers: Obesity raises the chances of developing cancers of the uterus, cervix, endometrial lining, cervix, breast, colon, rectum, esophagus, liver, gallbladder, pancreas, kidneys, and thyroid.

Gastrointestinal issues: Obesity raises the chances of developing heartburn, gallbladder disease, and liver issues.

Gynecological and sexual complications: Obesity in women can lead to infertility and irregular periods. Erectile dysfunction in men can also be caused by obesity.

Sleep apnea: Obese people are more likely to suffer from sleep apnea, a life threatening condition in which breathing repeatedly stops and starts while sleeping.

Osteoarthritis: Obesity raises the amount of stress exerted on weight-bearing joints while also causing inflammation in the body.

Intense COVID-19 symptoms: If you get infected with the virus that causes coronavirus disease, you're more likely to experience serious symptoms if you're obese (COVID-19). Serious cases of COVID-19 can necessitate treatment in intensive care units or even mechanical breathing assistance.

Quality of life: Obesity may have a negative effect on your overall quality of life. It's likely that you won't be able to do things you used to, such as engage in fun events. You may want to stop going to public places. Obese people can face prejudice as a result of their condition.

Other weight-related problems that may have an effect on your quality of life are:

- Anxiety
- Incapacity
- Sexual concerns
- Sad reflection and sorrow
- Isolation from others
- Poor Job productivity.

Prevention

You can take steps to avoid unhealthy weight gain and related health problems whether you're at risk of obesity, currently overweight, or at a healthy weight. Preventing weight gain is similar to preventing weight loss: daily exercise, a healthy diet, and a long-term commitment to watch what you eat and drink.

Exercise on a daily basis. To avoid weight gain, you can get 150 to 300 minutes of moderate-intensity exercise per week. Quick walking and swimming are examples of moderately vigorous physical activities.

Maintain a balanced eating schedule. Low-calorie, nutrient-dense foods, such as fruits, vegetables, and whole grains, should be prioritized. Limit your intake of saturated fat and candy, as well as alcohol. Eat three meals a day, with just a few snacks in between. As a special treat, you can also eat small quantities of high-fat, high-calorie foods. Simply make sure to eat foods that will help you maintain a healthy weight and overall health.

Recognize and prevent the food traps that contribute to overeating. Recognize the circumstances that lead to uncontrollable feeding. Write down what you eat, how often you eat, what you eat, how you're feeling, and how hungry you are in a diary. After a while, you can start to see trends. You should prepare ahead of time and devise strategies for dealing with these types of conditions while maintaining control over your eating habits.

Keep a close eye on your weight. People who weigh themselves at least once a week have a higher chance of losing weight. Monitoring your weight will tell you if your efforts are paying off and can help you spot minor weight gain before it becomes a major issue.

Consistency is essential. Sticking to your healthy-weight plan as much as possible during the week, on weekends, and during vacations and holidays increases the chances of long-term success.

Diagnosis for Obesity

A physical exam and other examinations are usually performed by the doctor to diagnose obesity.

These exams and tests typically include:

Taking your health history. Your doctor can inquire about your weight history, weight-loss attempts, physical activity and exercise habits, eating patterns and appetite management, previous medical conditions, medications, stress levels, and other health concerns. Your doctor can even look at your family's medical background and see if you're at risk for any illnesses.

A full physical test. Measuring your height, testing vital signs like heart rate, blood pressure, and temperature, listening to your heart and lungs, and inspecting your abdomen are all part of this process.

BMI (Body Mass Index) is a measurement of how healthy you are. Your BMI will be measured by your doctor (BMI). Obesity is described as a BMI of 30 or higher. The higher the number, the greater the risk to your health. Your BMI should be tested at least once a year to assess your overall health risks and potential therapies.

Measuring your waist circumference. Visceral fat, also known as abdominal fat, is fat accumulated around your abdomen that can increase your risk of heart disease and diabetes. Women with a waist circumference of more than 35 inches (89 centimeters) and men with a waist circumference of more than 40 inches (102 centimeters) may face greater health risks than those with smaller waist circumferences. Your waist circumference, like your BMI, should be tested at least once a year.

Testing for other health problems. Your doctor will assess any underlying health conditions you may have. Other potential health issues, such as high blood pressure and diabetes, will be checked by the doctor. Such heart checks, such as an electrocardiogram, may be recommended by your doctor.

Blood tests. The tests you undergo are dictated by your fitness, risk factors, and any current symptoms you might be experiencing. A cholesterol test, liver function tests, a fasting glucose test, a thyroid test, and other blood tests can be performed.

Gathering all of this knowledge will assist you and your doctor in deciding how much weight you need to lose as well as any potential health problems or risks. As a consequence, treatment decisions will be based on this knowledge.

Treatment

Obesity therapy aims to help people achieve and maintain a healthier weight. This increases your overall health and decreases your chances of developing obesity-related complications. To understand and improve your eating and exercise patterns, you will need to consult with a team of health professionals, including a dietitian, a behavioral psychologist, or an obesity specialist.

A moderate weight loss of 5% to 10% of your overall weight is normally the first treatment target. That means that if you weigh 200 pounds (91 kg) and have obesity according to BMI guidelines, you just need to lose 10 to 20 pounds (4.5 to 9 kg) to see a significant improvement in your health. The more weight you lose, though, the better.

Both weight-loss plans necessitate dietary modifications as well as increased physical activity. The treatment options that are best for you are determined by the magnitude of your obesity, your physical health, and your ability to follow through with your weight-loss plan.

DIETARY MODIFICATIONS

Obesity can be overcome by reducing calories and adopting healthy eating habits. While you can lose weight quickly at first, long-term weight loss is considered the best and most effective way to lose weight and keep it off permanently.

Avoid making dramatic and unrealistic dietary changes, such as crash diets, because they won't help you lose weight in the long run.

To increase the chances of weight loss success, commit to a rigorous weight-loss program for at least six months and at least a year in the maintenance process.

There is no such thing as the perfect weight-loss diet. Choose one that contains nutritious foods that you believe would be beneficial to you. Dietary changes to treat obesity include:

Eliminating calories. The trick to losing weight is to cut back on your calorie consumption. The first step is to assess your current eating and drinking habits and determine how many calories you consume on a regular basis and where you can make changes. To lose weight, you and your doctor will determine how many calories you need to eat per day, but a normal number is 1,100 to 1,500 calories for women and 1,500 to 1,800 for men.

Eating mindfully on less. Desserts, candies, fats, and processed foods, for example, have a lot of calories in a limited amount of food. Fruits and vegetables, on the other hand, offer a greater portion size with less calories. You will minimize hunger pangs, consume less calories, and feel better about your meal by consuming greater portions of lower-calorie foods, all of which contribute to how satisfied you feel overall.

Making better decisions. Eat more plant-based foods, such as fruits, vegetables, and whole-grain carbohydrates, to enhance your overall diet. Lean protein sources, such as beans, lentils, and soy, as well as lean meats, should be prioritized. If you like fish, make it a point to eat it twice a week. Regulate salt and added sugar. Consume small quantities of fats and ensure that they come from heart-healthy sources including olive, canola, and nut oils.

Restricting predefined foods. Some diets exclude certain food types, such as high-carbohydrate or high-fat foods. Inquire with your doctor about which diet plans have been shown to be successful and which would be beneficial to you. Sugar-sweetened drinks are a surefire way to eat more calories than you intended, so limiting or removing them is a good place to start when it comes to calorie reduction.

Meal substitutes. These diets recommend replacing one or two meals with their items, such as low-calorie shakes or meal bars, and eating healthy snacks and a nutritious, balanced third meal that is also low in fat and calories. This form of diet will help you lose weight in the short term. However, bear in mind that these diets are unlikely to teach you how to improve your overall lifestyle, so you will have to stick with it if you want to lose weight.

Fast fixes should be avoided. Fad diets that promise quick and easy weight loss can tempt you. However, the fact is that there are no miracle foods or fast fixes. Fad diets may help in the short term, but they don't seem to be any better in the long run than other diets.

Similarly, you can lose weight on a crash diet, but you will most likely gain it back once you quit. You must adopt healthy eating habits that you can sustain over time in order to lose weight — and keep it off.

PHYSICAL ACTIVITIES AND BENEFITS

Obesity therapy must involve increased physical activity or exercise. Most people who can keep their weight loss for more than a year exercise regularly, even if it's just walking.

To increase your level of operation, do the following:

Exercise: Obese people must engage in at least 150 minutes of moderate-intensity physical activity each week to avoid more weight gain or sustain a small weight loss. You will need to work-out for 300 minutes or more a week to see substantial weight loss. As your stamina and health improve, you'll possibly need to steadily increase the amount of exercise you do.

Keep on going: Even though frequent aerobic exercise is the most effective way to burn calories and lose weight, any additional movement aids in the process. Making small changes throughout the day can have a big impact. Parking farther away from store entrances, increasing household chores, gardening, getting up and moving around on a regular basis, and wearing a pedometer to track how many steps you take in a day are all good ideas. A good aim to set for yourself is to walk 10,000 steps per day. Increase the amount of steps you take to achieve your target gradually.

There are many types of physical activity, including swimming

- ✓ Running
- ✓ Jogging
- ✓ Walking
- ✓ Dancing etc.

Benefits of Regular Exercises
Active exercise has proven to have multiple physical and mental health benefits. It could encourage you to live longer.

This is how daily exercise helps your overall wellbeing.

✓   **It Will Make You Feel Happier.**

Exercise has shown that it improves mood and reduces depression, anxiety and fear. It results in changes in the brain that control stress and anxiety. It may also improve brain sensitivity for serotonin and norepinephrine hormones, which reduce depressed feelings.

Exercise can also increase the development of endorphins that are known to contribute to good emotions and the pain perception.

✓   **It Can Lead to Weight Loss.**

Most studies have shown that weight gain and obesity are caused by inactivity. The human body uses energy in three ways: digest food, exercise and manage the body's pulse and breathing functions. A decreased calorie intake during diet decreases the metabolic rate, thereby slowing weight loss. Normal activity has instead been demonstrated to improve your metabolic rate, allowing you to eat more calories and lose weight.

✓   **It's Indeed Good for Your Muscles and Bones.**

Exercise plays an important part in the development and maintenance of healthy bones and muscles.
23

Physical exercise like weight lifting, when combined with a sufficient amount of protein, will promote muscle building.

This is because exercise helps to release hormones that facilitate the absorption of amino acids by your muscles. This allows them to expand and decreases their collapse.

✓   **It Also Can Increase Your Energy Levels.**

Exercise can be a real boost of energy for stable individuals and people with different medical conditions. One research showed that weeks of daily training decreased tiredness in 20 healthy people with chronic tiredness. In fact, exercise in people with progressive disease, including cancer, HIV/AIDS and multiple sclerosis, has been shown to increase energy levels.

✓   **It May Reduce the Risk of Chronic Disease.**

A main cause of chronic illness is the lack of daily physical activity. Regular exercise has been shown to increase the sensitivity of insulin and cardiovascular health, thus lowering blood pressure and blood fat levels

✓   **It Will Help Your Brain Memory and Health.**

Exercise can enhance the function of the brain and protect memory and thinking skills.

First of all, it improves the heart rate that encourages blood and oxygen flow to your brain. It can also trigger hormone output that can improve brain cell development.

✓   **It Contributes to Rest and The Quality of Sleep.**

You can relax and sleep better with regular exercise. Another example was that the quality of sleep improved with 16 weeks of physical exercise and helped 15 people with insomnia sleep deeper and longer than the control group. During the day they even felt more energetic.

✓   **It Will Lessen Pain.**

Chronic pain can weaken, although exercise can help to alleviate it. Several studies have shown that exercise can help to control pain related to different health disorders, including chronic low back pain, fibromyalgia and chronic soft tissue shoulder disorder.

✓   **Can Improve Your Sex Life.**

Exercise was shown to stimulate sex

Regular exercise will boost the cardiovascular system, improve blood circulation, improve tone muscles and improve your sexual activity.

It also can boost the look of your skin, help you lose weight and keep it down, decrease chronic disease risk and enhance sex life.

Behavior changes

A behavior management program will assist you in making lifestyle changes and losing and sustaining weight loss. Examining your current behaviors to determine what causes, pressures, or situations could have contributed to your obesity are among the steps to take.

Everyone is different and faces different struggles when it comes to weight loss, such as a lack of workout time or late-night snacking. Make improvements to your actions that are specific to your issues.

The following are examples of behavior modification, also known as behavior therapy:

Counseling: Discussing with a mental health professional will help you cope with eating-related emotional and behavioral problems. Therapy will help

26

you understand why you overeat and how to deal with anxiety in a safe way. You can also learn how to keep track of your health and physical activity, recognize eating causes, and deal with food compulsions. Counseling may be done individually or in a group setting.

More rigorous plans: Such as those with 12 to 26 sessions a year, could be more effective in helping you meet your weight-loss goals.

Support groups: In community groups, where people face similar struggles with obesity, you will find camaraderie and empathy.

PRESCRIPTION WEIGHT-LOSS MEDICATION

A healthy diet and regular exercise are necessary for weight loss. Prescription weight-loss medication, on the other hand, may be helpful in some circumstances.

Remember that weight-loss medication should be used in conjunction with, not instead of, diet, exercise, and behavioral changes. Weight-loss drugs, also known as anti-obesity medications, help you adhere to a low-calorie diet by suppressing appetite and lack of fullness signals that arise while you're trying to lose weight.

If other diet and exercise programs have failed and you meet one of the following criteria, your doctor may recommend weight-loss medication.

27

If your BMI is 30 or higher, you're overweight.

You have a BMI of more than 27 and medical conditions associated with obesity, such as diabetes, high blood pressure, or sleep apnea.

Your doctor will assess your medical history as well as any potential side effects before prescribing a prescription for you. Some weight-loss drugs aren't safe for pregnant women, people who take those medications, or people who have chronic health problems.

Medications for treating overweight and obesity

Below are lists the medicines for weight loss approved by FDA. They include:

❖ **Phentermine-Topiramate:** the most active weight loss drug available today is the new release (Qsymia). It combines a neurostabilizer with an adrenergic agonist. Migraine and obesity adults are strong subjects for this drug.

Dose: 3.75/23mg – 15mg/92mg. daily.

Side effects include: uncontrolled sensations, lightheadedness, taste alterations, sleeplessness, constipation, and dry mouth.

Contraindications: Hypertension and heart disease, hyperthyroidism, glaucoma and stimulant sensitivity.

When weight loss of more than 5% is not attained after a maximum dose of 12 weeks, the weight loss pill should be phased out gradually.

❖ **Bupropion/Naltrexone (Contrave)**: incorporates a dopamine/norepinephrine reuptake inhibitor and an opioid receptor antagonist. It regulates food-related cravings and addictions.

Daily dose: 8/90 mg tablet – 4 tablets daily.

Side effects include: constipation, headaches, insomnia, and dry mouth.

Contraindications include: unmanaged hypertension, history of seizures, and opioid use and dependence.

❖ **Liraglutide (Saxenda)**: a GLP-1 receptor approved to use Victoza and Saxenda for diabetes type 2 and weight loss injection. Liraglutide delays digestion and causes feelings of fullness. Adults with diabetes and prediabetes are suitable candidates.

Dose: 0.6 mg – 3 mg daily.

Side effects include: nausea, vomiting, diarrhea, constipation, and stomach discomfort.

29

Contraindicated: patients with family history of medullary thyroid carcinoma.

❖ **Orlistat:** a pill that reduces weight which inhibits fat absorption in the gastrointestinal tract of pancreatic and gastric lipase. It can be taken together with food.

Daily dose: (120 mg Xenical) (60 mg Alli) (60 mg Alli).

Side effects include: diarrhea with fatty discharge and fecal urgency after consumption of high-fat foods.

Phentermine (Adipex, Ionamin, Suprenza) And Diethylpropion: oldest medications for weight loss. It was approved by FDA for short-term use and it is an adrenergic agonist that suppresses appetite

Daily dose: 15 mg – 37.5 mg (Lomaira).

Side effects include: dry throat, insomnia, blurry vision, and irritability.

Weight reduction drugs are just one part of a complex recovery plan for weight loss, it also includes dietary, physical activity, and behavioral therapies.

Note: Do not take these pills if you are pregnant or planning to. May lead to birth defects. Do not take if you are breastfeeding.

Tips On Medications for Weight Loss

- Follow the advice of your doctor on treatment for weight loss.
- Buy your medications from a doctor-approved pharmacy or online distributor.
- Take medicine for weight loss to sustain the physical and healthy eating plan.
- Know the side effects and precautions about any drugs.
- Ask your doctor if you can stop taking your medicine if after 12 weeks you do not lose weight.
- Speak to your doctor about other drugs, including supplements and vitamins, if you take weight loss medicines.
- Do not take weight-loss pills during pregnancy or if you expect to become pregnant.
- What medicines could work for me to lose weight?

You and your doctor should decide on a drug to treat overweight or obesity. Important factors are included:

- Possible weight loss benefits
- The potential side effects of the drug
- Your present health problems and other medications
- Your family's medical history
- Cost

How long does one need to take weight-loss medication?

It depends on whether the medicine helps you lose weight and maintain weight and whether you do have side effects. Talk to your doctor that if you have lost weight enough to improve your health, regardless of the side-effects. If, after 12 weeks of your medication, you do not lose at least 5% of your starting weight, your doctor will probably advise you not to take the medication. He or she can change your plan of treatment or think of another medication for weight loss.

WEIGHT-LOSS SURGERY

Weight-loss surgery, also known as bariatric surgery, is an option for certain people. Weight-loss surgery either restricts the amount of food you can consume safely or lowers food and calorie intake, or both. Although weight-loss surgery has the best chance of helping you lose the most weight, it also comes with a lot of risks.

Obesity surgery can be recommended if you have attempted and failed to lose weight by other approaches and:

You are morbidly obese (BMI of 40 or higher)

You have a BMI of 35 to 39.9 and a severe weight-related health condition, such as diabetes or high blood pressure. You're determined to make the lifestyle changes needed for surgery to be successful.

Some people will lose up to 35 percent or more of their excess body weight with weight-loss surgery. However, weight-loss surgery isn't a cure-all for obesity.

It does not ensure that you will lose any of your extra weight or that you will be able to hold it off in the long run. Your ability to lose weight after surgery is contingent on your willingness to make long-term improvements in your diet and exercise habits.

Common weight surgeries include:

Gastric bypass surgery. The surgeon produces a small pouch at the top of your stomach during gastric bypass (Roux-en-Y gastric bypass). The small intestine is then cut and attached to the new pouch a short distance below the main stomach. Food and liquids drain straight from the pouch into this section of the intestine, bypassing the stomach for the most part.

- **Adjustable Gastric Banding**:

An inflatable band is used to split the stomach into two pouches during this process. The surgeon establishes a tiny channel between the two pouches by pulling the band close like a belt. The band prevents the opening from widening and is intended to remain in place indefinitely.

- **Duodenal Switch and Biliopancreatic Diversion**:

The surgeon will start by extracting a large portion of the stomach. The valve that releases food into the small intestine and the first portion of the small intestine are left alone by the surgeon (duodenum). The surgeon then closes off the middle portion of the intestine and connects the last section to the duodenum directly. To allow bile and digestive juices to flow into this portion of the intestine, the separated section is reattached to the end of the intestine.

- **Gastric Sleeve**:

A portion of the stomach is eliminated in this process, resulting in a smaller food pool. Compared to gastric bypass or biliopancreatic diversion with duodenal switch, it's a less daunting treatment.

Other Treatments

Obesity may also be treated with vagal nerve blockade. It entails implanting a system underneath the abdominal skin that sends irregular electrical signals to the abdominal vagus nerve, which informs the brain when the stomach is empty or complete. This new technology was approved by the FDA in 2014 for adults with a BMI of 35 to 45 and at least one obesity-related disease, such as type 2 diabetes, who have not been able to lose weight with a weight-loss program.

Preventing Weight Regain After Treatment

Unfortunately, no matter what obesity treatment strategies you try, you're likely to gain weight again. When you avoid taking weight-loss pills, you'll almost certainly gain weight. If you continue to overeat or overindulge in high-calorie foods or drinks after weight-loss surgery, you can also gain weight.

Regular physical exercise is one of the easiest ways to stop regaining the weight you've lost. Aim for 45 to 60 minutes of exercise a day.

If it encourages you stay focused and on track, log your physical activity. Speak to your doctor about what new things you may be able to do as you lose weight and improve your health, and, if possible, how to increase your activity and exercise.

It's possible that you'll have to keep an eye on your weight for the rest of your life. The easiest way to maintain the weight you've lost off in the long run is to incorporate a healthy diet with more exercise in a realistic and sustainable manner.

Take it one day at a time when it comes to weight loss and maintenance, and surround yourself with positive tools to help you excel. Find a healthy lifestyle that you can maintain in the long run.

HOME REMEDIES AND A HEALTHY LIFESTYLE

If you adopt methods at home in addition to your formal treatment plan, your attempt to combat obesity is more likely to succeed. This may involve the following:

Learning more about your condition.

Obesity education will help you understand why you've become obese and what you can do about it. You may feel more confident in your ability to take charge and adhere to your treatment plan. Read reputable self-help books and talk with your doctor or therapist about them.

Setting attainable objectives.

When you need to lose a lot of weight, you can set unrealistic targets, such as trying to lose too much weight too quickly. Don't put yourself in a position to fail. Set exercise and weight-loss targets for yourself on a daily or weekly basis. Make incremental changes to your diet rather than trying to make dramatic changes that you won't be able to maintain in the long run.

Following your treatment plan.

Changing a lifestyle that you've been living with for a long time can be challenging. If you note that your exercise or diet goals are slipping, notify your doctor, therapist, or other health care providers. You should collaborate to come up with new approaches or concepts.

Recruiting support.

Encourage your family and friends to join you in your weight-loss efforts. Surround yourself with people who can promote and assist you rather than hinder your efforts. Ascertain that they are aware of the importance of weight loss to your wellbeing. Joining a weight-loss support group can also be beneficial.

Keeping track.

Holding a diet and activity journal is a smart idea. This journal will help you stay on track with your diet and exercise habits. You will figure out what behaviors are holding you back and, conversely, what behaviors work well for you. You may also use your journal to keep track of other vital health indicators including blood pressure, cholesterol, and overall fitness.

Food triggers must be recognized and prevented. Abstain yourself from the need to eat by doing something constructive, such as calling to a friend. It's a good idea to get in the habit of saying no to unhealthy foods and large portions. Eat because you're hungry, not because the clock says it's time to eat.

Taking your drugs exactly as prescribed.

If you're taking a weight-loss drug or one to treat obesity-related conditions like high blood pressure or diabetes, follow the instructions carefully. Speak to your doctor if you're having trouble sticking to your prescription schedule or if you're experiencing adverse side effects.

Medicines that may not be conventional

There are several dietary supplements on the market that claim to help you lose weight quickly. These products' efficacy, especially long-term effectiveness, and safety are frequently questioned.

The Food and Drug Administration classifies herbal medicines, vitamins, and minerals as dietary supplements, which are not subjected to the same stringent monitoring and labeling as over-the-counter and prescription drugs.

However, some of these substances, including "natural" products, have drug-like effects that can be harmful. When taken in excess, even certain vitamins and minerals can create issues. Ingredients could be substandard, resulting in unexpected and potentially harmful side effects. Dietary supplements can also interfere dangerously with any prescription drugs you're taking. Before taking any dietary supplements, consult your doctor.

Acupuncture, mindfulness therapy, and yoga are examples of mind-body approaches that can be used in conjunction with other obesity treatments. However, these therapies haven't been extensively researched in the treatment of obesity. If you're interested in adding a mind-body therapy to your care, talk to your doctor.

Coping and Assistance.

✓ **Keep a log**: To express pain, rage, anxiety, or other emotions, keep a journal.

✓ **Connect**: Don't separate yourself. Make an effort to engage in regular events and catch up with family or friends on a regular basis.

✓ **Join**: Join a support group to meet people who are going through similar situations.

✓ **Focus**: Maintain your attention on your objectives. Obesity recovery is a long-term operation. Keep your goals in mind to stay inspired. Remind yourself that you are in charge of handling your condition and achieving your objectives.

✓ **Allow yourself to unwind**: Learn how to relax and control the tension. Learning to identify stress and practicing stress management and relaxation techniques may aid in the maintenance of unhealthy eating habits.

Preparing for Your Appointment

One of the most important things you can do for your wellbeing is to share your weight issues with your doctor frankly and honestly. In some cases, you may be referred to an obesity specialist — if one is available in your area. A behavioral psychologist, dietitian, or nutrition consultant may be assigned to you.

What you can do to help

It's important that you take an active role in your treatment. Preparing for your appointment is one way to do this. Consider the medical conditions and priorities. Make a list of questions to ask as well. The following are examples of possible questions:

- ✓ What diet and exercise habits are most likely to blame for my health problems and weight gain?
- ✓ What should I do about the difficulties I'm having with weight management?
- ✓ Do I have any other health issues as a result of my obesity?
- ✓ Is it necessary for me to see a dietitian?
- ✓ Do I see a behavioral therapist who specializes in weight loss?
- ✓ What are my choices for treating obesity and my other health issues?
- ✓ Is a weight-loss program for me a viable option?

Make sure your doctor is aware of any medical conditions you may be suffering from, as well as any prescription or over-the-counter medications, vitamins, or supplements you are taking.

What would you expect from your doctor?

Your doctor will likely ask you a series of questions about your weight, eating habits, physical activity, mood and emotions, as well as any symptoms you might be experiencing during your appointment. You could be asked questions like:

- ✓ When you were in high school, how much did you weigh?
- ✓ What life events may have contributed to your weight gain?
- ✓ In a normal day, what do you eat and how much do you eat?
- ✓ In a typical day, how much operation do you get?

- ✓ What were the times in your life that you gained weight?
- ✓ What factors do you think influence your weight?
- ✓ How does your weight affect your day-to-day life?
- ✓ What weight-loss diets or therapies have you tried?
- ✓ What weight-loss targets do you have in mind?
- ✓ Are you willing to make lifestyle changes in order to lose weight?

✓ What factors do you believe are preventing you from losing weight?

In the meantime, there are a few things you can do.

If you have time until your scheduled appointment, you can help yourself prepare by keeping a diet diary for two weeks prior to the appointment and using a step tracker to track how many steps you take each day (pedometer).

You should also start making decisions that will help you lose weight, such as:

✓ **Make lifestyle changes that are beneficial for you**. Increase the intake of fruits, vegetables, and whole grains. Reduce the scale of your portions.

✓ **Increasing your level of physical activity**. Make an effort to get up and walk around your house more often. If you aren't in good shape or aren't used to exercising, begin slowly. Even a daily 10-minute walk will help. If you have any health problems or are over a certain age — over 45 for men and 55 for women — wait to start a new fitness program until you've spoken with your doctor.

Foods to Eat

The following are examples of foods to eat:

- **Vegetables**: Asparagus, collard greens, peppers, spinach, Brussels sprouts, broccoli, kale, watercress, beets, tomatoes, cauliflower, etc.
- **Fruits**: Blueberries, blackberries, pomegranate, oranges, star fruit, strawberries, watermelon, cantaloupe, guava, tangerines, apples, etc.
- **Carbs**: Sweet potato, plantains, beans, quinoa, lentils, potatoes, maize, amaranth, nonfat refried beans, brown rice, edamame, peas, buckwheat, etc.
- **Proteins**: Sardines (fresh or canned), skinless chicken or turkey breast, egg whites, fish (cod, salmon, tuna, tilapia, catfish, trout), whole eggs, tofu, etc.
- **Hearty fats**: Almonds, walnuts, peanuts, hummus, pistachios, cashews, pecans, avocados, coconut milk and cheeses (, parmesan, goat, feta).
- **Seeds and dressings**: Sunflower seeds, pumpkin seeds, olives, sesame seeds, ground flax seeds etc.
- **Oils and nut butter**: Extra-virgin olive oil, extra-virgin coconut oil, pumpkin-seed oil, flaxseed oil, walnut oil, nut butter (peanut, almond, cashew, etc.) seed butter (sunflower, pumpkin, tahini) etc.
- **Seasonings and condiments**: Lemon or lime juice, ginger, spices, garlic, mustard, herbs, vinegar (cider, white wine, or red wine), etc.

- **Recommended beverages**: Water, coffee, green tea, fruit-infused water, sparkling water and unsweetened iced tea.

Trigger Foods to Avoid

When following Beachbody nutrition programs, the following are not recommended:

Added sugars: Sweetened beverages, baked goods, sweetened yogurts, candy, table sugar, etc.

Refined carbs: White pasta, bagels, sugary cereals, white bread, tortillas, white rice, corn chips etc.

Processed foods: Fast food, energy bars, packaged snacks, (hot dogs, deli meats, bacon), canned foods packed in syrup, processed meats, etc.

Greasy and fried foods: Fried chicken, burgers, pizza, French fries, deep-fried foods, potato chips etc.

Alcohol: Liquor, wine, beer etc.

OBESITY IN CHILDREN

One third of children in the United States are overweight or obese and this figure tends to rise Children have less health and medical conditions related to weight than adults. Overweight children, however, are at high risk of being overweight

45

teenagers and adults, putting them at risk for developing chronic conditions later in life, such as heart disease and diabetes. Obese children are more likely to be mocked or harassed by their peers. This can lead to a decrease in self-esteem as well as an increased risk of mental health and depression.

Causes Obesity in Children
Obesity in children is caused by a combination of lifestyle factors, inadequate physical activity, and an excess of calories from food and beverages. However, genetic and hormonal factors can also play a role.

Many causes, most of which work in concert, raise your child's risk of being overweight:

- **Diet**: Eating high-calorie foods on a regular basis, such as fast food, baked goods, and vending machine snacks, can lead to weight gain in your kid. Candy and sweets can also lead to weight gain, and there is growing evidence that sugary beverages, such as fruit juices and sports drinks, are to blame for certain people's obesity.

- **Lack of physical activity**: Since they don't burn as many calories as children who exercise regularly, they are more likely to gain weight. Sedentary habits such as watching television or playing video games add to the issue as well. Ads for unhealthy foods are often shown on TV shows.

- **Family factors**: Your child will be more likely to gain weight if he or she comes from a family of people who are obese. This is particularly true in a setting where high-calorie foods are readily available and physical activity is demotivated.

- **Psychological factors**: Social, parental, and family stress may all contribute to a child's obesity risk. Some children eat junk to cope with difficulties or feelings like stress, or to prevent boredom. It's likely that their parents have similar tendencies.

- **Socioeconomic factors**: Some people in some areas have restricted resources and supermarket access. As a result, they can opt for shelf-stable convenience foods like frozen meals, crackers, and cookies. Additionally, people who live in lower-income areas may lack access to a safe place to exercise.

- **Certain medications**: Some prescription medications have been related to an increased risk of obesity. Prednisone, lithium, amitriptyline, paroxetine (Paxil), gabapentin (Neurontin,

Gralise, Horizant), and propranolol (Propranolol) are among them.

Risk Factors of Obesity in Children

Obese children are at risk for a variety of factors, such as:

- High cholesterol
- High blood pressure
- Early cardiac condition
- Diabetes
- Bone concerns
- Skin disorders such as heat rash, bacterial infections and acne

Checking If Your Child Is Overweight

Your child's doctor is the right person to verify whether your child is overweight or not. If your child is overweight, the doctor measures the weight and the height of your child and calculates the "BMI" to compare it with standard. The doctor will also examine at the age and trends of growth of your child.

Supporting an Overweight Child

It is really important that your child knows you are supportive, especially when they are overweight. Children's sensations about themselves are always focused on the emotions of their parents and they would be more likely to feel good about themselves if parents accept them with some weight. It is important to discuss their weight with your children so that they can share their concerns with you. Your child's doctor will also assist you in defining healthy weight objectives for the height of your child. The doctor may also instruct you on a schedule for healthy BMI.

Parents should not distinguish children due to their weight. Parents should instead concentrate on the physical activity and eating habits of their families. Everyone is taught good habits by including the whole family.

Tips for Healthy Habits
There are several ways to get the whole family interested in healthy habits, but increasing physical activity is particularly important. Tips include:

Set a good example. Your children will be more likely to be healthy and remain active for the rest of their lives if they see you being physically active and having fun.

- Plan family events that everybody will participate in, such as walking, biking, or swimming.

- Be aware of your child's needs. Children who are overweight can feel self-conscious about engaging in some activities. It's necessary to assist your child in finding physical activities that they enjoy which aren't too frustrating or humiliating.

- Reduce the amount of time you and your family spend doing sedentary hobbies like watching television or playing video games.

- Make healthy meals together as much as possible, and shop for healthy foods together.

- Improving the whole family's food and exercise habits is one of the most effective ways to eliminate childhood obesity. Childhood obesity can be treated and prevented, which helps to protect your child's health now and in the future.

When to See a Doctor

Consult your child's doctor if you're concerned that he or she is gaining too much weight. Your child's growth and development history, your family's weight-for-height history, and where your child falls on the growth charts will all be taken into account by the doctor. This can help you figure out if your child's weight is unhealthy or not.

BMI percentile range	Category
below 5th percentile	Underweight
5th to 84th percentile	Healthy weight
85th to 95th percentile	Overweight
Above 95% percentile	severe obesity

Since BMI doesn't take into consideration things like muscle mass or a larger-than-average body frame, and because children's growth patterns vary so much, your doctor will take into account your child's development and growth. This can help you figure out if your child's weight is a health issue.

Treatment of Obesity in Children
Treatment for childhood obesity is determined by the age of your child and whether he or she has any other medical conditions or not. Changes in your child's eating habits and level of physical activity are typically part of the care. In certain cases, medicine or weight-loss surgery may be used to treat the disease.

Procedure for children with BMIs between the 85th and 94th percentiles (overweight)

The American Academy of Pediatrics suggests that overweight children over the age of two be placed on a weight-maintenance program to slow the rate of weight gain. This technique helps the child to gain inches but not pounds, resulting in a BMI that falls into a healthy range over time.

Treatment for children who have a BMI of 95 percentile or higher (severe obesity)

Children aged 6 to 11 who are obese will be advised to change their eating habits in order to lose no more than 1 pound (0.5 kilogram) each month. Obese or severely obese older children and adolescents may be encouraged to change their eating habits in order to lose up to 2 pounds (or about 1 kilogram) per week.

The strategies for sustaining or losing weight in your child are the same: your child must eat a balanced diet — both in terms of food type and quantity — and increase physical activity. Your dedication to assisting your child in making these improvements is vital to his or her progress.

WEIGHT-LOSS SURGERY IN CHILDREN WITH OBESITY

Adolescents with extreme obesity who have been unable to lose weight by lifestyle changes may be candidates for weight-loss surgery. However, there are uncertainties and long-term complications associated with this form of surgery. Talk to your child's doctor about the benefits and drawbacks.

If your child's weight poses a greater health risk than the surgery's risks, your doctor may recommend this procedure. A team of pediatric experts, including an obesity medicine consultant, a psychologist, and a dietitian, should consult with the child who is considering weight-loss surgery.

Surgery for weight loss isn't a cure-all. It does not ensure that an adolescent can lose weight or be able to hold it off in the long run. Surgery also doesn't take the place of a balanced diet and daily exercise.

Coping and Assistance

Parents are key to making children feel loved and in control of their weight. Make the most of any chance to raise your child's self-esteem. Don't be afraid to bring up the subject of fitness and health. Directly, frankly, and without being negative or judgmental, speak to your children.

In addition, try the following:

53

Avoid weight discussion. Even if well-intentioned, derogatory remarks about your own, someone else's, or your child's weight may hurt your children. Negative weight talk can lead to an unfavorable body image. Instead, talk about healthy food and having a good body image.

Dieting and skipping meals should be avoided. Instead, promote and endorse increased physical activity and healthy eating.

Find ways to compliment your child on his or her efforts. Tiny, subtle improvements in behavior should be celebrated, but not with food. Some choices for celebrating your child's milestones include going to the bowling alley or a nearby park.

Discuss the child's emotions with him or her. Assist your child in coping with feelings in ways other than eating.

Assist your child in focusing on constructive objectives. For instance, mention that he or she can now ride a bike for more than 20 minutes without tiring out or that he or she can now run the specified number of laps in gym class.

Patience is required. Recognize that a laser-like focus on your child's eating habits and weight can easily backfire, leading to even more overeating or the development of an eating disorder.

Getting Ready for Your Appointment

The initial diagnosis of childhood obesity would most likely be made by your child's family doctor or pediatrician. If your child's obesity causes complications, you might be referred to additional specialists to help handle these issues.

Questions to bring up with your doctor

If possible, bring a friend or family member with you to help you remember everything you learn. Some specific questions to ask your doctor about childhood obesity include:

- ✓ What other health concerns is it possible that my child will face?
- ✓ What treatment options are available?
- ✓ Are there any medications that could help my child manage his or her weight and other health issues?
- ✓ How long would it take to complete the treatment?

✓ What should I do to assist my child in burning fat?
✓ Do you have any brochures or other printed materials that I could have? What are some of your favorite websites?

Don't be hesitant to ask other questions.

What to expect from your specialist?

Your child's doctor or other health care professional is likely to ask you a series of questions about his or her dietary habits and physical activity, such as:

✓ In a normal day, what does your child eat?
✓ In a normal day, how much activity does your child get?
✓ What do you think influences your child's weight?
✓ Which, if any, diets or therapies have you sought to assist your child in losing weight?
✓ Are you willing to make lifestyle changes in your family to assist your child in losing weight?
✓ What might be obstructing your child's weight loss efforts?
✓ How often does your family eat as a unit? Is the child involved in the food preparation?
✓ Is it normal for your child or family to eat while watching TV, texting, or working on a computer?

In the meantime, there are a few things you can do.

Keep track of what your child eats and how involved he or she is in the days or weeks leading up to his or her scheduled appointment.

OBESITY IN PREGNANT WOMEN

When you're pregnant, it's critical to eat enough to provide your growing baby with the nutrients he or she needs to thrive. Most doctors advise pregnant women to gain a little weight, but what should you do if you're already overweight?

Obese women are more likely to experience pregnancy complications including preeclampsia and gestational diabetes. Premature birth and such birth defects are often more likely in their infants. In the past, doctors were hesitant to encourage obese women to lose weight during pregnancy for fear of harming the baby. However, recent research indicates that obese women can safely exercise and eat to lose weight without jeopardizing their baby's health.

You can still have a good pregnancy and delivery if you're obese. Continue reading for advice on how to lose weight safely and successfully when pregnant.

Losing Weight While Expecting a Child

Obese women who received diet and exercise therapy during their pregnancy had better results for both mother and baby, according to a new report. The women were instructed on how to eat a well-balanced diet, keep a food journal, and engage in light physical activity such as walking.

These interventions, especially dietary changes, were linked to a 33 percent lower risk of preeclampsia and a 61 percent lower risk of gestational diabetes, according to the report. Healthy eating has decreased the risk of gestational hypertension and premature births. If you're obese and expecting a child, your pregnancy might be the ideal time to kick-start a healthier lifestyle.

Complications of Obesity During Pregnant

Obesity raises your chances of having complications while pregnant. The higher your BMI, the more likely you are to develop the following conditions:

- Miscarriage is a common occurrence in women.
- Gestational diabetes
- Preeclampsia and high blood pressure
- Clots in the blood
- After the birth, there was more bleeding than normal.

Obese or not, these issues will affect any pregnant woman. However, as the BMI rises, the danger rises as well.

Complications of Obesity for Unborn Babies
Obesity can also put your baby at risk for health issues.

The following are possible issues for your baby:

- Early birth (before 37 weeks)
- Increased birth weight
- Excess body fat at birth
- Spina bifida and other birth defects
- Stillbirth

Later in life, you're more likely to develop a chronic illness such as heart disease or diabetes.

Losing Weight During Pregnancy
All you do should be done in moderation. Now is not the time to try a rigid fad diet or a rigorous workout regimen.

Consult Your Specialist

Before starting an exercise program while pregnant, consult your doctor. They will assist you in creating a routine and provide answers to any questions you might have. Your doctor may also refer you to a dietitian or trainer for an assessment and tailored advice on healthy eating and exercise while pregnant.

Take Advantage of Your Pregnancy

Pregnancy is an excellent time to begin an exercise regimen and make dietary improvements. Pregnant women are more likely than non-pregnant women to see their doctor often and ask a lot of questions. They are also more likely to make lifestyle changes in order to keep their baby healthy.

Begin slowly.

Any new exercise should be started slowly and gradually increased over time. Start with five or ten minutes of exercise a day. The next week, add five minutes more.

Your ultimate aim should be to stay active for 30 to 45 minutes a day. For people who are new to fitness, walking and swimming are also excellent options. They're both kind to the joints.

✓ Keep a journal

Keeping a food journal is an excellent way to ensure that you're getting enough nutrients and water each day. You will find out whether the diet contains too much sugar or sodium, or whether it is deficient in a certain nutrient. A journal can also be used to keep track of your mood and appetite.

Furthermore, keeping a journal is the most effective way to prepare your workout schedule and develop a routine that fits you. It's best if you can get into a routine as soon as possible.

There are numerous community forums where you can connect with others who share your goals. You may also share exercise plans, recipes, and other useful hints for sustaining your new healthy lifestyle.

✓ **Stay away from empty calories.**

Eat and drink in moderation (or completely avoid) the following foods and beverages during pregnancy:

- Fast food
- Fried food
- Microwave dinners
- Soda
- Pastries
- Desserts

Dietary improvements were found to be more successful than exercise alone in helping women lose weight and boost their baby's outcomes. The women followed a well-balanced diet that included a variety

61

of carbohydrates, proteins, and fats, as well as keeping a food log to ensure they were getting enough nutrients.

✓ Shun fad diets

It's not a good idea to try a new diet during your pregnancy. These diets are generally low in calories. They won't give your baby the nutrients he or she needs to remain healthy. Diet fads, on the other hand, can be extremely risky for your baby if they cause you to lose weight too fast or limit your food choices. Your baby needs a variety of vitamins that he or she cannot obtain from a restricted diet. It's preferable to think of it as a lifestyle modification rather than a diet.

✓ Don't Overwork Yourself

Physical activity of a moderate intensity will not harm your baby. Strenuous exercise, on the other hand, can be risky during pregnancy. A good rule of thumb is that while exercising, you should be able to comfortably carry on a conversation with a friend. If you can't talk because you're breathing so heavily, you're probably working out too hard. Pay attention to the body. Stop working out and take a rest if anything hurts.

Skiing, horseback riding, and mountain biking are all examples of contact sports or activities that can throw you off balance and cause you to fall. If you want to cycle, a stationary bicycle is safer than a regular bike.

Prenatal Supplements Are Recommended

While a healthy, balanced diet provides the majority of the vitamins and minerals you and your unborn child require, a prenatal supplement can help fill in the gaps. Adult multivitamins are not the same as prenatal vitamins. They have more folic acid, which helps to prevent neural tube defects, as well as more iron, which helps to prevent anemia.

Since your body will not feel deprived, prenatal supplements may help you prevent cravings and overeating.

You can have a successful pregnancy even though you're overweight. Maintain a healthy lifestyle by staying active and eating nutritious foods. The number on the scale is less important than giving your baby the vitamins and nutrients he or she requires. If you can't lose weight, don't worry. Just keep eating healthy and exercising moderately, and try to avoid gaining weight.

When you get your baby home, continue to eat and workout so that you can be a healthy mother.

HEALTHY EATING MEAL PLAN FOR BEGINNERS: A 14-DAY WEIGHT LOSS MEAL PLAN (1,200 CALORIES)

If you're new to a clean meal, it is straightforward — but you can easily understand what it's all about by following a meal plan. Clean food is an excellent way to increase your consumption of nutritious foods (such as whole grains, lean protein, healthy fats and a lot of fruits and veggies) while limiting the trigger foods such as calories, alcohol, added sugars and hydrogenated fats.

This simple weight loss meal plan includes all organic foodstuffs and limits refined foodstuffs to help you regain your healthy habits.

If you feel like you have fallen short of your good habits, this easy clean-up will help you regain a feeling for the best food. During this 14-day diet, you can get your nutritious food filling. Some are prepared from scratch and others you can purchase from the shop.

You'll feel energized, fulfilled and happy about what's on your plate through the meals and snacks on this plan. This diet meal plan will set you to lose up to 4 pounds over two weeks with 1200 calories.

WEEK 1

Preparing Your meals for the Week

A little planning at the beginning of the week makes the rest of the week very enjoyable.

Prepare Greek Meatball Mezze Bowls to serve for lunch on 2nd day till the 5th day. Keep fresh for the week in an air-tight bag.

Prepare Lemon-Tahini Dressing double batch. You'll eat it for lunch and dinner during the week. Keep your salad dressing in this vintage glass bottle.

Cook a big batch of Easy Brown Rice to last you the whole week. Store in a large glass food container. Since the Kale Salad with Beets & Wild Rice on Day 1 calls for wild rice, you can either make a larger batch or substitute brown rice in the recipe to avoid having to make 2 kinds of rice.

DAY 1

Breakfast (285 calories)

- Muesli and Raspberries (1 serving)

Tip: While purchasing muesli, opt for a brand that does not contain added sugars, as these sugars detract from the health benefits of this whole-grain breakfast.

Morning Snack (62 calories)

• 1 medium orange

Lunch (359 calories)

• Salad with White Beans and Veggies (3 cups)

Snack at 5:00 p.m. (94 calories)

• 1 medium apple

Dinner (419 calories)

• Kale Salad with Beets and Wild Rice, 4 cups (1½ servings)

• 1 serving Chicken Balsamic-Dijon

Daily Stats: 1,219 calories, 61 g protein, 153 g carbohydrates, 40 g fiber, 47 g fat, 1,400 mg sodium.

DAY 2

Breakfast (269 calories)

• Avocado-Egg Toast (1 serving)

Shopping Tip: Sprouted-grain bread, unlike many store-bought breads, is made without added sugars, so use it as your bread for the next two weeks. Also, if you're going to use hot sauce to top your egg toast, look for a brand that doesn't have any added sugars.

Morning Snack (100 calories)

• 1 medium pear

Lunch (391 calories)

• 1 serving Mezze Bowl with Greek Meatballs

Snack at 5:00 p.m. (61 calories)

• 1 medium orange

Dinner (438 calories)

• Squash & Red Lentil Curry (1 serving cup)

• ½ cup Easy Brown Rice

Daily Stats: 1,221 calories, 63 g protein, 147 g carbohydrates, 33 g fiber, 46 g fat, 1,965 mg sodium.

DAY 3

Breakfast (286 calories)

• Muesli with Raspberries (1 serving)

Morning Snack (61 calories)

• 1 medium orange

Lunch (391 calories)

• Mezze Bowl with Greek Meatballs (1 serving)

Snack at 5:00 p.m. (91 calories)

• 12 almonds

Dinner (438 calories)

• 1 serving Asian Tilapia with Green Beans (Stir-fried)
• 1 cup Easy Brown Rice

Daily Stats: 1,201 calories, 62 g protein, 174 g carbohydrates, 37 g fiber, 48 g fat, 1,444 mg sodium.

DAY 4

Breakfast (256 calories)

• 1½ cup cooked rolled oats in 1 cup milk

• 1 chopped medium plum

Meal-Prep Tip: Cook oats and serve them with a plum and a pinch of cinnamon on top.

Morning Snack (95 calories)

• 1 apple, medium

Lunch (391 calories)

• 1 serving Mezze Bowl with Greek Meatballs

Snack at 5:00 p.m. (105 calories)

• 1 banana, medium

Dinner (431 calories)

• 1 serving Chicken on a Sheet Pan with Brussels Sprouts

• 1 ½ cup mixed greens with 2 tbsp. lemon-tahini dressing

Daily Stats: 1,209 calories, 58 g protein, 166 g carbohydrates, 32 g fiber, 41 g fat, 1,553 mg sodium.

Day 5

Breakfast (287 calories)

• 1 serving Cinnamon Toast and Peanut Butter with Bananas

Shopping tip: Avoid store-bought peanut butter products with added sugars and trans fats while shopping for a nutritious snack. More information on selecting a good peanut butter can be found here.

Morning Snack (31 calories)

• ½ cup raspberries

Lunch (391 calories)

• Mezze Bowl with Greek Meatballs (1 serving)

Dinner (542 calories)

• Pork Chops with Garlicky Broccoli (1 serving)

Daily Stats: 1,220 calories, 54 g protein, 102 g carbohydrates, 30 g fiber, 71 g fat, 1,175 mg sodium.

DAY 6

Breakfast (258 calories)

• ½ cup cooked rolled oats in 1 cup milk

• 1 chopped medium plum

Meal-Prep Tip: Cook oats and serve them with a plum and a pinch of cinnamon on top.

Morning Snack (102 calories)

1 medium pear

Lunch: (326 calories)

• Veggie & Hummus Sandwich (1 serving)

 Shopping Tip: Review the ingredient list on hummus to make sure it doesn't have any added sugars or sodium. You may even make your own.

Snack at 5:00 p.m. (63 calories)

• 1 medium orange

Dinner (544 calories)

• Butternut Squash Rice-Stuffed Peppers (1 serving)

• 2 cups mixed greens with 1 tablespoon dressing Citrus Vinaigrette.

Meal-Prep Tip: Save the rest of the Citrus Vinaigrette for the next meal.

Daily Stats: 1,208 calories, 57g protein, 146 g carbohydrates, 31 g fiber, 49 g fat, 1,120 mg sodium.

DAY 7

Breakfast (306 calories)

• 2 cups Avocado Green Smoothie by Jason Mraz

Morning Snack (34 calories)

• 1 clementine

Lunch (351 calories)

• Lettuce, Cucumber, and White-Bean Salad with Basil Vinaigrette (2 ¼ cup)

• 1 toasted slice of sprouted-grain bread with 1 tbsp. hummus

Tip: Save a serving of the Tomato, Cucumber, and White-Bean Salad with Basil Vinaigrette for 10th Day's lunch. Store the dressing properly and separately.

Snack at 5:00 p.m. (29 calories)

• 1 plum

Dinner (489 calories)

• 1½ cups Mexican Cabbage Soup

• 2 cups No-Cook Black Bean Salad

Meal-Prep Tip: preserve 1-cup serving of the No-Cook Black Bean Salad for lunch on 9th Day. Store the dressing apart and wait until ready to eat. In a leak-proof bag, pack 2 servings of the Mexican Cable Soup

73

Daily Stats: 1,209 calories, 35 g protein, 163 g carbohydrates, 48 g fiber, 55 g fat, 1,365 mg sodium.

WEEK 2

Preparing Your meals for the Week

A little planning at the start of the week can make your remainder simple.

Make an invitation to prepare the Greek Kale salad with quinoa & chicken recipe for dinner on 8 Day, using the Meal-Prep Sheet-Pan Chicken Thigh and Basic Quinoa. This way, during the week you can use residual chicken and quinoa. Big glass meal-prep containers store the rest of the chicken and quinoa separately.

DAY 8

Breakfast (338 calories)

• Scrambled Eggs with Vegetables (1 serving)

Morning Snack (119 calories)

• ¼ cup hummus

• 1 cup cucumber slices

Lunch (325 calories)

• Veggie & Hummus Sandwich (1 serving)

Snack at 5:00 p.m. (30 calories)

• 1 plum

Dinner (302 calories)

• Greek Kale Salad with Quinoa and Chicken (serves 1)

Evening Snack (102 calories)

• 1 serving Broiled Mango

Daily Stats: 1,216 calories, 58 g protein, 121 g carbohydrates, 26 g fiber, 60 g fat, 1,816 mg sodium.

DAY 9

Breakfast (306 calories)

• 2 cups Jason Mraz's Avocado Green Smoothie

Morning Snack (34 calories)

• 1 clementine

Lunch (327 calories)

• 1 ½ cup Cabbage Soup (Mexican)

• 1 cup No-Cook Black Bean Salad

Snack at 5:00 p.m. (91 calories)

• ¾ cup Kiwi & Mango with Fresh Lime Zest

Dinner (452 calories)

• 1 cup rice cauliflower, heated

• 1 serving Soy-Lime Roasted Tofu

• 2 cups Colorful Roasted Sheet-Pan Veggies

• 1 Tbsp. Citrus Vinaigrette

Toss the riced cauliflower with the tofu, veggies, and vinaigrette.

Daily Stats: 1,211 calories, 44 g protein, 149 g carbohydrates, 42 g fiber, 59 g fat, 1,248 mg sodium.

DAY 10

Breakfast (289 calories)

• Peanut Butter-Banana Cinnamon Toast (1 serving)

Morning Snack (63 calories)

1 cup raspberries

Lunch (369 calories)

• 1 serving Apple Kale Wraps with Chicken

Snack at 5:00 p.m. (91 calories)

• 1 plum

• a pound of almonds

Dinner (401 calories)

• Asian Slaw with Panko-Crusted Pork Chops (1 serving)

Daily Stats: 1,212 calories, 72 g protein, 127 g carbohydrates, 29 g fiber, 50 g fat, 1,133 mg sodium.

DAY 11

Breakfast (269 calories)

• Avocado-Egg Sandwich (1 serving)

Morning Snack (63 calories)

1 pound raspberries

Lunch (301 calories)

• Greek Kale Salad with Quinoa and Chicken (serves 1)

Snack at 5:00 p.m. (94 calories)

• 1 apple, medium

Dinner (477 calories)

• Lemon-Garlic Butter Sauce with Salmon and Asparagus (1 serving)

• 1 cup Quinoa (Basic)

Meal-Prep Tip: Cook a hard-boiled egg tonight so it'll be ready for your P.M. Snack on Day 12.

Daily Stats: 1,204 calories, 68 g protein, 128 g carbohydrates, 28 g fiber, 50 g fat, 1,233 mg sodium.

DAY 12

Breakfast (289 calories)

• Cinnamon Toast with Peanut Butter and Bananas

(1 serving)

Morning Snack (95 calories)

• 1 clementine

• a pound of almonds

Lunch (343 calories)

• 1 ½ cup Cabbage Soup (Mexican)

• ½ cup cups mixed greens

• 1 tablespoon vinaigrette (citrus)

• sunflower seeds, 2 tbsp.

Preparation:

In a large mixing bowl, toss the greens with the vinaigrette. Sunflower seeds are sprinkled on top.

Snack at 5:00 p.m. (77 calories)

• 1 hard-boiled egg, finely seasoned with salt and pepper

Dinner (407 calories)

• Spaghetti Squash & Meatballs (1 serving)

Daily Stats: 1,211 calories, 60 g protein, 124 g carbohydrates, 30 g fiber, 56 g fat, 1,463 mg sodium.

DAY 13

Breakfast (263 calories)

• 1 cup plain Greek yogurt (nonfat)

• a quarter cup of muesli

• a quarter cup of blueberries

Morning Snack (69 calories)

• 2 clementine

Lunch (324 calories)

• Veggie & Hummus Sandwich (1 serving)

Snack at 5:00 p.m. (94 calories

• 1 apple, medium

Dinner (445 calories)

• 1 serving Zucchini Noodles with Shrimp and Avocado Pest

Daily Stats: 1,195 calories, 68 g protein, 133 g carbohydrates, 31 g fiber, 52 g fat, 1,102 mg sodium.

DAY 14

Breakfast (269 calories)

• 1 serving Avocado-Egg Toast

Morning Snack (69 calories)

• 2 clementine

Lunch (377 calories)

• Tomato, Cucumber, and White-Bean Salad with Basil Vinaigrette (2 ½ cup)

• 1 toasted slice sprouted-grain bread with 2 tbsp. hummus

Snack at 5:00 p.m. (29 calories

• 1-pound plum

Dinner (457 calories)

• 1 serving Coconut-Shallot Sauce Fish

• ¼ cup Quinoa (Basic)

• 2 tsp citrus vinaigrette on 2 cups mixed greens

Daily Stats: 1,202 calories, 61 g protein, 113 g carbohydrates, 27 g fiber, 60 g fat, 1,146 mg sodium.

You did it!

You did a great job sticking to this balanced eating schedule. We hope you find this diet plan inspiring, entertaining, and informative, whether you made every single recipe in it or not. Keep up the good work, and don't forget to check out some other nutritious meal plans.

125 HEALTHY AND EFFECTIVE WEIGHT LOSS RECIPES AROUND THE GLOBAL

Slow Cooker Seafood Ramen

Ingredients:

- 1 lb. seafood
- 64 oz. broth (seafood, vegetable, or chicken • 4–6 oz. ramen
- 2 tablespoons low sodium soy sauce
- 1 teaspoon salt
- ½ lb. tomatoes, sliced
- 2 green onions, sliced
- 2 tablespoon rice vinegar
- 2 garlic cloves, minced
- 1/4 cup kale, chopped
- 1/8 teaspoon red pepper flakes
- 1/4 teaspoon sesame oil

- 1/4 teaspoon pepper

Directions:

Step 1

Put all the ingredients except seafood, kale and ramen into the slow cooker. Stir well.

Step 2

Cook on high heat for 2-3 hours, or cook on low heat for 4-6 hours.

Step 3

Add seafood and kale and cook for 15 minutes

Per Serving: 247 calories, 2.7 g fat (0.3 g sat), 29.5 g protein, 26 g carb, 258 mg sodium, 3 g sugars, 1.6 g fibre

Turkey Carrot Mushroom Dumplings

Ingredients:

- lb. ground turkey
- 1/2 cup mushrooms finely chopped
- 30 dumpling
- tsp soy sauce
- ¾ c. carrots finely julienned
- 1 teaspoon rice wine

- 1/2 teaspoon onion powder
- 1 teaspoon sesame oil
- 1/8 teaspoon salt
- teaspoon corn-starch

Directions:

Step 1

Put the carrots in a microwave bowl and cover the pot with water. Cook until tender, about 5 minutes, depending on how fine the carrots are cut. Drain and cool.

Step 1

In a large bowl, mix the cooked carrots, turkey, mushrooms, soy sauce, rice wine, sesame oil, onion powder, salt and corn-starch. Stir well.

Step 3

Put one tablespoon of round filling on the dumpling wrapper. Seal and fill with wrapping paper. Wrap the remaining dumplings

Step 4

Boil the water at the bottom of the steamer. Place the dumplings in a steamer lined with parchment paper. Steam for 15 minutes until cooked.

Per serving: 56 calories, 2 g fat (0 g sat.), 3 g protein, 6 g carb, 87 mg sodium

Slow Grilled Chinese Char Siu Chicken

Ingredients:

- 1/4 cup organic ketchup
- 1/4 cup raw honey
- Cooking oil spray
- ¼ c. organic brown sugar
- 1/4 cup gluten-free soy sauce
- 3 tablespoon beet powder
- 1 tablespoon gluten-free hoisin sauce
- 2 1/2 lbs. boneless skinless chicken thighs
- 2 tablespoon rice vinegar
- ½ teaspoon Chinese five-spice powder • Sea salt and freshly ground black pepper to taste

Directions:

Step 1

In a large bowl, mix brown sugar, honey, ketchup, soy sauce, beet powder, vinegar, sea scent sauce, allspice, salt and pepper.

Step 2

Mix the chicken well, cover all the pieces and Refrigerate for two days to marinate.

Step 3

Heat the grill, spray cooking oil on the stove oil, grill the chicken until cooked, about 10 minutes each time.

Per serving: 328 calories, 7 g fat (2 g sat), 38 g protein, 26 g carb, 846 mg sodium, 24 g sugars, 1 g fibre

Creamy Kabocha Squash and Roasted Red Pepper

Ingredients:

- 1 small kabocha squash
- 1 head of garlic
- • 1/3 cauliflower, cut into large florets
- ½ cup raw cashews
- 1/2 medium onion (roughly chopped)
- 1 medium carrot, roughly chopped
- 1 stalk celery, roughly chopped

- 1/4 c. roasted red peppers, drained
- 2 tablespoon nutritional yeast
- A pinch red pepper flakes (optional)
- Salt and black pepper, to taste
- 1/2 to 3/4 c. fresh basil (unpacked), sliced
- 2 to 3 c. vegetable broth (or as needed)
- 2 lb. gluten-free spaghetti noodles (or pasta of your choice)

Serve with:

- Fresh basil, sliced
- Black pepper
- Vegan parmesan cheese (optional)

Directions*:*

Step 1

Soak cashew nuts in water all through the night, if you don't have time, you can boil water and add cashew nuts. Let them soak, then mix the sauce together (about 1 hour).

Step 2

Preheat the oven to 400°F, then place the rack in the middle of the oven. Line a baking sheet with parchment paper or silicone mat.

Step 3

Wash and dry the kabocha squash, place it (whole) on a baking sheet and place in the oven for 18-20 minutes. Remove the pan from the oven and cool until the squash is easy to handle. If its rod protrudes, use a knife to carefully remove it.

Step 4

Cut the pumpkin in half vertically, and scoop out the seeds and fibre with a spoon. Cut the pumpkin into 1-inch wedges to make the slices even and even cook.

Step 5

Place 6 or 7 slices of cooked pumpkin (about 1 ½ cups) on a lined baking sheet. Leftover kabocha squash can be cooked on other baking sheets. It can be stored in a container in the refrigerator for up to a week.

Step 6

Use your hands to remove the loose skin on the outside of the garlic head. Use a sharp knife to cut ¼ inch from the garlic head, or fully expose the top of the clove. Place the garlic (cut side down) on the baking sheet along with the broccoli florets, onions, celery and carrots. Sprinkle with salt and pepper, return to the oven for 35 minutes, flip/mixing halfway through. 10 minutes before the vegetables are done, prepare the pasta.

Step 7

Once the roasting pan is removed from the oven, cool the vegetables to be easy to handle, and then carefully remove the skin from the kabocha with a knife and add it to the high-speed mixer. You can discard it or snacks while you continue cooking. With your hands.

Step 8

Squeeze the softened garlic cloves from the head, put them in a blender, pour the cashew nuts (drained), the remaining vegetables on the baking tray, roasted red pepper, nutritional yeast, red pepper flakes, 2 cups of vegetable soup with salt and pour into the blender and pepper base on needs. Mix until smooth and add an extra 1 cup of vegetable broth as needed to make the sauce thin. Season with seasonings, then add chopped basil.

Step 9

Pulse basil until well mixed (don't mix it, because it will turn the sauce into a weird colour). Drain the pasta, put it back in the pot, and pour it over the sauce. Mix until well mixed then sprinkle with fresh Parmesan cheese, basil and black pepper. Enjoy your meal

Per serving: 311 calories, 6 g fat (0 g sat), 17.8 g protein, 83.4 g carb, 46.3 mg sodium, 5.8 g sugars

Loaded Cauliflower
Ingredients:

- 6 green onions, chopped into the green and white parts
- 2 tablespoon butter
- 1.25 lb. cauliflower head, cut into florets
- 3 garlic cloves, minced
- 2 oz. cream cheese
- 1/4 teaspoon black pepper
- 3/4 cup organic heavy whipping cream
- 2 c. cheddar cheese, grated
- 1.5 teaspoon ranch seasoning Mix, optional
- ½ teaspoon sea salt
- Olive oil for roasting the cauliflower
- 4 slices sugar-free bacon, crumbled
- Dollops of sour cream, optional

Directions:

Step 1

Preheat the oven to 420 degrees, pour the cauliflower and 2 tablespoons of olive oil into the pot, then add it to the baking dish. Roast the cauliflower on the baking sheet for 20 minutes. Cauliflower will become tender and some parts will be brown.

Step 2

While roasting the cauliflower, season the cheese, add the butter, scallion and garlic cloves to a frying pan over medium heat. Fry until the onion is translucent (3 minutes) then put the cream cheese, salt, ranch seasoning (if used) and pepper together with the onion, garlic and butter in a frying pan.

Step 3

Reduce the heat to a medium level and continue to cook until the cream cheese melts. Stir in 1.5 cups of cheddar cheese to complete the cheese sauce.

Step 4

Mix the cheese sauce and roasted cauliflower, then add it to the baking dish. Put the remaining cheddar cheese on top and bake for another 20 minutes until the cauliflower is tender. then put roasted cauliflower on top, some sour cream, green parts of spring onions and chopped bacon on top.

Per serving: *315 calories, 25 g fat (17 g sat), 12 g protein, 8 g carb, 597 mg sodium,*
2 g sugars, 1 g fibre

Easy Creamy Cajun Shrimp Pasta

Ingredients:

- 2 teaspoons olive oil Divided into 1 teaspoon servings.
- 1 tablespoon Cajun seasoning divided into ½ tablespoon servings. (You can also use creole seasoning)
- 1 lb. raw shrimp, deveined and shells removed.
- 8 oz. linguine pasta
- 4 oz. andouille sausage Sliced into 1inch pieces.
- 1/2 cup chopped red peppers
- 1/2 cup chopped green peppers
- 1/2 cup chopped yellow or white onions
- 1 tablespoon butter
- 1/2 cup heavy whipping cream
- 1/2 cup unsweetened almond milk
- 1 c. fire roasted diced tomatoes, drained from a can.
- 4 oz. cream cheese Cut into chunks.
- 1/2 c. shredded Parmesan Reggiano Cheese

Directions:

Step 1

Cook the pasta as per package instructions.

Place the shrimp in a bowl along with 1/2 tablespoon of Cajun or creole seasoning. Mix to ensure the shrimp is fully coated.

Step 2

Heat a skillet or pan on medium high heat. Use a cast iron skillet then add 1 teaspoon of olive oil to the pan, when hot, add the shrimp to the pan. Cook for 3 minutes on each side until it turns bright pink, remove the shrimp and set aside add an additional teaspoon of olive oil to the pan along with the chopped sausage, onions, green peppers and red peppers.

Step 3

Sauté for 4 minutes until the vegetables are soft and the onions are translucent and fragrant. Remove the vegetables from the pan and set aside.

Step 4

Reduce the heat on the pan to medium. Add the butter to the pan and allow it to melt, add in the heavy cream, almond milk, cream cheese, the remaining 1/2 tablespoon of Cajun or creole seasoning, and parmesan Reggiano cheese, continue to stir the sauce until all of the cheese has fully melted. The cream cheese may take some time to melt.

Step 5

Add in the fire roasted tomatoes and stir. Allow the mixture to cook for 2-3 minutes then add the shrimp, sausage, vegetables, and pasta to the pan and stir. Allow the pasta to cook for 4-5 minutes until combined. Serve.

Per serving: 364 calories, 27 g fat, 7 g protein, 22 g carb

Healthy Chicken Taco Soup

Ingredients:

- 1 small yellow onion diced
- 1 small red bell
- pepper, diced
- ½ tablespoon avocado or coconut oil
- 1 small green bell pepper, diced
- 5 cloves garlic, minced
- 1 lb. boneless, skinless chicken breast
- 1 teaspoon dried oregano
- 1 teaspoon chipotle powder
- 1 ½ teaspoon salt (plus more to taste)
- 1 teaspoon paprika
- 2 teaspoon cumin
- ¼ teaspoon black pepper
- 1 – 15 oz. can fire roasted diced tomatoes
- 2 – 4.5 oz. cans green chilies
- ¼ c. fresh lime juice
- Cilantro, for serving

- Diced red onion, for serving
- 32 oz. chicken broth
- Lime wedges, for serving

Directions:

Step 1

Heat a large pot over medium heat. After heating, add avocado or coconut oil. Next, add the peppers, onions and garlic to the pot. Fry until the onion starts to become translucent.

Step 2

Add chicken breast, canned tomatoes, canned green peppers, spices, lime juice and chicken broth to the pot. Stir well. Bring the soup to a boil, then reduce the heat to low heat. Boil the soup for 30 minutes or until the chicken is tender and easy to shred.

Step 3

Move the chicken breast from the soup to a bowl, use two forks to chop the meat.

Step 4

Pour the chicken into the soup and stir until fully combined. Serve the soup with fresh cilantro, diced red onion and fresh lime cubes. Enjoy your meal.

Quick and Easy Mongolian Beef

Ingredients:

- 2 tablespoon corn-starch
- 2-4 tablespoon canola oil
- 1 lb. Flank steak thinly sliced against the grain
- 1 yellow onion sliced
- 4 garlic cloves chopped
- 1-inch ginger chopped
- ¼ c. Water
- ¼ c. Low sodium soy sauce
- 2 green onions chopped, green and white parts separated
- 3 tablespoon brown sugar
- 1 tablespoon hoisin sauce
- Salt to taste

Directions:

Step 1

Cover the hind legs with corn-starch, making sure that each piece is covered. Set aside. Heat the canola oil in a large pot at medium high temperature. Once the oil is hot, add the flank steak in a single layer to the frying pan, making sure it is not touching, cook for 2-3 minutes on each side until brown on both sides. Cook in batches until all flank steaks are cooked. Set aside.

Step 2

Cover the thinly sliced yellow onion, green onion, garlic and ginger on the frying pan and stir-fry until the onion is slightly soft but still a bit chopped then you put the soy sauce, water, hoisin sauce and brown sugar then stir.

Step 3

Pour the steak and the green part of the onion into the pot. Remove from the heat and eat.

Per serving: 308 calories, 15 g fat (3 g sat), 26 g protein, 20 g carb, 680 mg sodium, 11 g sugars, 1 g fiber

Caribbean Steamed Fish

Ingredients:

- Juice of 1 lime
- ½ teaspoon black pepper
- 1 teaspoon salt
- 2 lbs. fish (porgy or snapper), cleaned and scaled
- 15 sprigs thyme
- ½ Tablespoon butter
- ½ Tablespoon oil
- 3 cloves garlic – 2 sliced and 1 crushed
- 2 carrots, thinly sliced
- 1 red pepper, thinly sliced
- 1 green pepper, thinly sliced
- 1 onion, thinly sliced
- 1 hot pepper (scotch bonnet, habanero or wiri wiri), seeds removed
- 12 okras, ends cut off
- 1 ½ cup water

Directions:

Step 1

Season the fish with lime juice, minced garlic, black pepper, salt and half of thyme and set aside.

Step 2

In a large, wide, thick-bottomed pot, heat over medium heat, add oil and butter. After the butter has melted, sauté the carrots, red and green peppers and onions until they become soft in about 5 minutes, then add garlic flakes and pepper and cook for a minute or two.

Step 3

Add water to boil. Pour the fish into the pot. Scoop some vegetables on the fish. Add the okra and the rest of the thyme.

Step 4

Cover the pot and cook on low heat, then cook for 15 minutes, until cooked. Remove from the heat and eat.

Per serving: *378 calories, 7.4 g fat (1.2 g sat), 60.5 g protein, 13.1 g carb, 794 mg sodium, 5.5 g sugars, 3.3 g fiber.*

Corn Chowder Con Chile Poblano

Ingredients:

- 1 poblano pepper without seeds and thinly sliced
- 2 cloves of garlic roughly chopped

- 5 corn husks
- 1 medium onion sliced
- 2 tablespoon vegetable oil
- 4 medium potatoes cubed
- 1 teaspoon of salt
- Corn kernels
- Pumpkin seeds
- Cilantro microgreens or chopped cilantro
- Olive oil
- Freshly ground pepper

Directions:

Step 1

Put oil and sliced poblano chili in a large pot. Put it there until it starts to soften, then add onion and garlic, and let stand for 5 minutes, or until the onion is found to be translucent, then add corn kernels, potatoes, salt and cover with water, then add salt and you cover. Let stand for 15 minutes or until the vegetables are cooked.

Step 2

Use a ladle to add about one-third of the vegetables and liquid to the container of the blender, mix until completely liquefied and fully integrated, then put the rest of the vegetables back into the pot. You can add some water if it's needed then check the seasoning and adjust if necessary.

Step 3

Serve with drizzle olive oil, pumpkin seeds, corn kernels, sprouts or chopped coriander. Finally add sea salt and pepper.

Per serving: 138 calories, 4 g fat (3 g sat), 4 g protein, 24 g carb, 303 mg sodium, 1 g sugars, 4 g fibre

Crispy Potato Tacos

Ingredients:

- 1 c. mashed potatoes
- 4 tablespoon of vegetable oil or avocado oil
- Thinly sliced romaine
- Radishes thinly sliced
- 12 corn tortillas
- 4 long wooden skewers
- lettuce or green cabbage
- Cilantro
- Guacamole
- Salsa Verde

Directions:

Step 1

Place the tortillas on a frying pan and heat for 15 seconds to make them flexible, then place a spoonful of mashed potatoes in the centre of each tortilla and spread it along the tortillas, roll the tortillas and place them on long skewers.

Step 2

Repeat the above steps until 3 or 4 tortillas are placed on the baking pan repeat this for all tortillas.

Step 3

Put a tablespoon of oil in a high temperature frying pan, then add 3 or 4 tortillas for 5 minutes until golden brown, then turn to the other side.

Step 4

Take out the tacos and put them in paper towels to absorb the excess oil, repeat until all tacos are made.

When eating, put the crispy potato tacos on the plate and finish the toppings. Enjoy.

Per serving: 327 calories, 18 g fat (2 g sat), 6 g protein, 47 g carb, 31 mg sodium, 1 g sugars, 4 g fiber

Black Garlic, Sesame and Shitake Cod

Ingredients:

- 2 Alaskan Cod filets, frozen
- 1 teaspoon sesame seeds
- 2 tablespoons olive oil
- 1 clove black garlic
- ½ c. dried shiitake, rehydrated

Directions:

Step 1

Preheat the oven to 450°F. Rinse the frozen fish, pat dry with a paper towel, and place on a non-stick pan

Step 2

In a small bowl, add black garlic and heat in the microwave for 10 seconds.

Step 3

Mash the garlic cloves, then add olive oil and sesame seeds, brush this mixture on the frozen fish fillets, then sprinkle the mushrooms around the fish and put the fish in the oven for 15 minutes according to the thickness of the fish. If the fillet is thicker, turn it over during cooking

Step 4

Serve with rice, your favourite salad or whole grains.

Per serving: 221 calories, 13.8 g fat (2.1 g sat), 20 g protein,
6.1 g carb, 72 mg sodium, 1.2 g sugars,
1 g fiber

Shrimp Lettuce Wraps

Ingredients:

- 1 tablespoon hoisin sauce
- 1 teaspoon rice
- Vinegar
- ½ tablespoon low-sodium soy sauce
- ¼ c. Low-sodium chicken broth
- ¼ teaspoon Asian sesame oil
- 1 head butter lettuce or romaine lettuce hearts
- 1 1/2 teaspoon chili garlic sauce
- ½ teaspoon corn starch
- 1 tablespoon canola or avocado oil divided
- 30 grams' cashews little less than ¼ cup, coarsely chopped
- ⅛ c. Chopped cilantro
- 6 oz. shrimp deveined & cut into small cubes
- 1/2 large red bell pepper seeded and diced

- 1 carrot shredded or cut into thin strips
- 3 green onions the white and green parts, sliced
- 1 large garlic clove minced

Directions:

Step 1

Cut the lettuce into leaves and set aside.

Step 2

In a small bowl, stir together chicken broth, hoisin sauce, soy sauce, rice vinegar, sesame oil, chili garlic sauce and corn starch. Set aside

Step 3

In a medium frying pan, heat a tablespoon of rapeseed oil or avocado oil over medium heat until you almost smoke then add shrimp and fry until brown. Transfer the shrimp to the plate for about 2 minutes, and then remove the juice from the pan.

Step 4

In the same frying pan, heat another tablespoon of oil over medium heat, add garlic, sweet pepper, green onion and carrot then fry until crispy for about 2 minutes then return the shrimp to the pot, add cashew nuts and coriander.

Step 5

Add the soy sauce mixture and stir fry until the shrimp is fully cooked.
About 3 minutes pour the shrimp mixture evenly on the lettuce leaves.

Per serving: 249 calories, 16 g fat (2 g sat), 26 g protein, 18 g carb, 623 mg sodium, 8 g sugars, 3 g fiber

Easy Vegetable Stir-fry with Peanut Sauce

Ingredients:

Peanut Sauce:

- 1/4 teaspoon garlic powder (2 cloves)
- 3 tablespoons low sodium soy sauce
- 1/2 c. Smooth unsweetened peanut butter
- 1 tablespoon sesame oil
- ½ teaspoon ground ginger (1 tablespoon fresh)
- 2 tablespoons freshly squeezed lime juice
- 2 tablespoon maple syrup
- 1 tablespoon rice vinegar
- 2 tablespoons fresh lime juice
- 1/4 cc-1/3 cc water as needed
- Sriracha, to taste (optional)

- 3 cloves garlic, finely minced
- 1 tablespoon freshly grated ginger
- 6 oz. dried noodles of choice
- 1 tablespoon cooking oil of choice
- 1/3 c. Shredded red cabbage
- 4 oz. Crimini mushrooms, sliced
- 2 tablespoon green onions sliced
- 1 medium carrot, thinly sliced
- 1 c. Broccoli
- 2 large handfuls fresh baby spinach
- 1 medium red bell pepper, thinly sliced

Garnish:

- Cilantro, finely chopped
- Toasted sesame seeds or crushed peanuts
- 1 large lime, sliced
- Green onions, sliced

Directions:

Step 1

Prepare peanut butter in a small pot in a medium-low, add sesame oil, garlic and ginger cook until fragrant, add the remaining peanut butter ingredients and stir well. Simmer the mixture for a while, then remove it from the heat and set it aside.

Step 2

Prepare the noodles according to the package instructions. After the noodles are cooked, drain them, rinse them with cold water, put them back in the pot, and mix with about 1 teaspoon Sesame oil to prevent adhesion meanwhile, enlarge the wok over medium heat then add cooking oil, garlic, shallots and ginger. Stir-fry, stirring often for 3 minutes or until fragrant then add cabbage, mushrooms, carrots, bell peppers and broccoli. Cook for another 4 minutes.

Step 3

After the vegetables are cooked, add spinach, peanut butter and cooked noodles, mix until everything is well mixed, and cook for another 2 minutes until everything is cooked

Step 4

Serve with coriander, green and toasted sesame seeds, and add extra lime juice on the side. Enjoy your meal

Per serving: 368 calories, 18.7 g fat, 8.7 g protein, 48 g carb, 274.5 mg sodium, 11.6 g sugars

Grilled Chicken and Vegetable Shish Kebabs

Ingredients:

- 2 lb. boneless chicken breasts
- 1 whole zucchini
- 2 Tablespoon Better Than Bouillon roasted chicken base
- 8 oz. cubed pineapples
- 1 red bell pepper
- 2 teaspoon oregano
- 1 green bell pepper
- 2 teaspoons paprika
- 1 orange bell pepper
- 2 teaspoons black pepper

Teriyaki pineapple sauce:

- 2 teaspoon Sesame Oil
- 2 teaspoon minced garlic
- ¼ teaspoon Himalayan salt
- 2 Tablespoon fresh pineapple juice
- ½ c. low-sodium soy sauce
- 2 tablespoon brown sugar
- 2 teaspoon corn starch
- 1 teaspoon black pepper
- 1/4 teaspoon garlic powder

Directions:

Step 1

First set a fire on the grill to bring the temperature to 340 degrees.

Step 2

Cut the chicken breasts into small cubes and put them in a large bowl, season the chicken with oregano, black pepper and paprika, then rub the ingredients into the chicken then add better than Bouillon roasted chicken base to the chicken mix well together and set aside.

Step 3

Remove the stem and seeds from each sweet pepper and cut into large pieces. Cut the zucchini into thin slices.

Put each ingredient on the skewers in the required order. Put each chicken and vegetable skewers on the grill. Bake on each side for 4 minutes then remove from heat

Step 4

For soy sauce, put all the ingredients in a small pot on medium/high heat until it starts to bubble, then slow down and cook for 7 minutes, then remove from heat and cool. Serve hot.

Per serving: 428 calories, 5 g fat (0.4 g sat), 56.7 g protein, 35 g carb, 1268 mg sodium, 22.2 g sugars, 3.9 g fiber

Easy Baked BBQ Seitan

Ingredients:

- 1 teaspoon garlic powder
- 2 tablespoon nutritional yeast
- 1 c. vital wheat gluten
- 2 teaspoons smoked paprika
- 1 tablespoon soy sauce
- 2 tablespoon tahini
- 2 teaspoon onion powder
- 1 c. veggie broth
- 1/3 c. BBQ sauce of choice

Directions:

Step 1

Preheat the oven to 320°F. Add the wheat gluten, garlic powder, nutritional yeast, smoked paprika, and onion powder to a bowl, and mix with a fork to make sure it is well mixed.

Step 2

Add soy sauce, sesame paste and vegetable soup, then stir with a fork and mix the liquid into the flour until it forms a dough-like dough.

Step 3

Knead the gluten ball gently with both hands a few times to make sure not to over-mix. It should not exceed one minute.

Step 4

Transfer the dough to a lined baking pan. Flatten the dough and spread it out until the thickness reaches half an inch. Put the baking sheet in the oven for 30 minutes, then remove seitan from the oven and brush both sides with your favourite barbecue sauce. At this stage, you can grill or re-bake seitan.

Step 5

Put seitan in the oven for another 10 minutes. You can also choose to roast on high heat for about 3-4 minutes to help add a little charcoal to the ends of the seitan

Step 6

Place seitan on a preheated electric grill and cook or sear each side for about 5 minutes, or until grill marks appear on the surface of the seitan, once the seitan is placed on a clean surface or plate, let it sit for 3-5 minutes, then cut and use.

Per serving: 132 calories, 3.6 g fat (0.6 g sat), 12 g protein, 12.6 g carb, 534 mg sodium, 4.8 g sugars, 2.5 g fiber

Broiled Tilapia with Thai Coconut Curry Sauce

Ingredients:

- 1 Tablespoon minced peeled fresh ginger
- 1 teaspoon dark sesame oil, divide
- 4 garlic cloves, minced
- 1 c. chopped scallions
- 1 teaspoon curry powder
- 2 teaspoons red curry paste
- 1 c. finely chopped red bell pepper
- 1 Tablespoon brown sugar
- 2 teaspoon Asian fish sauce
- ½ teaspoon ground cumin
- 1 14-oz. can light coconut milk
- 4 teaspoon low-sodium soy sauce, use tamari for gluten-free
- 6-oz tilapia fillets
- ¼ c. chopped fresh cilantro
- Salt

Directions:

Step 1

Preheat the broiler. Heat the teaspoon of oil in a large pot over medium heat add ginger, garlic, pepper and green onions, cook for 2 minutes. Stir curry powder, curry paste and cumin; cook for 1 minute

Step 2

Add soy sauce, sugar, Asian fish sauce and coconut milk (do not cook). Remove from the heat.

Step 3

If necessary, stir the coriander or basil, brush the fish with 1 teaspoon of oil and sprinkle with a teaspoon of salt. Place the fish on a baking sheet coated with cooking spray.

Step 4

Boil for 7 minutes, or until the fish easily peels off when tested with a fork.

Serve the fish with the sauce, rice and lime wedges.

Per serving: 226 calories, g fat (0 g sat), 32.5 g protein, 4.6 g carb, 1.1 g fiber

Crockpot Beef Vegetable Soup

Ingredients:

- 1 lb. boneless chuck roast or beef stew meat — cut into • 1-inch cubes
- 1 Tablespoon extra-virgin olive oil
- ¼ teaspoon black pepper
- 2 teaspoons kosher salt, divided
- 1 small yellow onion, diced
- 3-4 c. low sodium beef broth — divided
- 2 cloves garlic — minced (about 2 tsp)
- 4 large carrots — peeled and finely chopped
- 2 parsnips — peeled and diced
- 2 ribs celery — diced
- 1 14.5-ounce can dice tomatoes
- 1 can tomato sauce (8 ounces)
- 2 Yukon gold potatoes — peeled and diced
- 3 Tablespoon tomato paste
- 1 Tablespoon Worcestershire sauce
- 1 teaspoon dried oregano
- ½ teaspoon smoked paprika
- ½ teaspoon granulated sugar
- Chopped fresh parsley — optional for serving
- 1 c. peas — fresh or frozen (no need to thaw)

Directions:

Step 1

In a large frying pan, heat oil over medium heat, then add beef, sprinkle with a teaspoon of salt and pepper. Make all sides of the beef brown and disturb it as little as possible on each side to make it a beautiful colour. After the beef is light brown (not fully cooked), move it to a 6-quart slow cooker then cook until the onions start to soften.

Step 2

Add garlic and stir for 20 seconds Sprinkle about ½ cup beef broth and scrape off any brown crumbs sticking to the bottom (this is the taste). Let the broth reduce for 3 minutes, then transfer the entire mixture to a slow cooker.

Step 3

To the slow cooker add carrots, potatoes, parsnips, celery, diced tomato juice, ketchup, ketchup, Worcestershire, oregano, paprika, sugar, 2 ½ cups beef broth and the remaining 1 teaspoon of salt.

Step 4

Cover the pot and cook for 8 hours, until the beef and vegetables are tender. Stir the peas until hot. If the remaining 1 cup of beef broth is thicker than needed, you can add it until it reaches the desired level. Serve hot and sprinkle with fresh parsley.

Per serving: 253 calories, 7 g fat (2 g sat), 23 g protein, 24 g carb, 12 g sugars, 8 g fiber

Sheet Pan Turkey Meatloaf and Broccoli Ingredients:

- 6 Tablespoon ketchup, divided
- 1.3 lb. (20 oz.) 93% ground turkey
- ⅓ c. minced onion
- 1 large egg
- ⅓ c. quick cooking oatmeal, or gf oats
- ¾ teaspoon kosher salt
- teaspoon kosher salt
- teaspoon Worcestershire sauce, divided
- 1 large bunch broccoli, (1 ½ pounds) cut into florets
- ½ teaspoon dried or fresh thyme leaves
- 2 Tablespoon olive oil

Directions:

Step 1

Preheat the oven to 430F. Line a 13x9-inch pan with Reynolds wrapped non-stick aluminium foil, with the food side facing down.

Step 2

In a medium-sized bowl, add broccoli oil and seasonings to taste with teaspoon salt, then on the flat bottom Spread out one side of the pan in a single layer then add turkey, oatmeal, tomato sauce, onion, egg, teaspoon salt, one teaspoon Worcestershire sauce and thyme in a bowl, and mix well, divide the mixture into 4 equal parts. Shape each part into a 4 x 3 inch free-form bread and place it on the other side of the pan.

Step 3

In a bowl, mix the remaining 2 tablespoons of tomato paste with the remaining 1 teaspoon of Worcestershire sauce, Spread on the bread.

Step 4

Bake in the oven for 20 minutes in the centre of the oven. Rotate the broccoli halfway until the meat is cooked in the middle, then slightly char the broccoli.

Per serving: 245 calories, 15 g fat (4 g sat), 35 g protein, 23.5 g carb, 753 mg sodium, 4 g sugars, 6g fiber

Blackened Chicken Cobb Salad

Ingredients:

- ¾ teaspoon paprika
- ¾ teaspoon garlic powder
- ½ teaspoon sea salt
- 1 tablespoon olive oil (if needed)
- ¼ teaspoon pepper
- pinch of cayenne pepper
- ¾ teaspoon chili powder
- 12 c. baby spinach or chopped romaine
- 1 lb. boneless skinless chicken breasts (3–4 pieces)
- 1 c. grape tomatoes, halved
- 1 large cucumber, sliced
- 1 c. baby Bella mushrooms, sautéed
- ½ c. red onion, chopped
- 1–2 avocados, sliced
- 4 large eggs, hard-boiled, peeled and sliced
- 6 slices cooked turkey bacon, crumbled
- ½ c. crumbled blue cheese (optional)

Ingredients for the red wine vinaigrette:

- ⅓ c. red wine vinegar
- 1 tablespoon Dijon mustard
- ¾ teaspoon sea salt
- 1 teaspoon maple syrup or honey

- ½ teaspoon black pepper
- ½ c. extra virgin olive oil

Directions:

Step 1

Beat the chicken dry with paper towels, then add chili powder, garlic powder, chili powder, sea salt, black pepper and chili powder in a small bowl. Spread the spice mixture on each chicken breast.

Step 2

When cooking, you can grill it on the indoor or outdoor grill, or on the stove, add 1 tablespoon of olive oil to the large frying pan over medium heat. Put the chicken breast in the hot oil, cook for about 7 minutes on each side until the juice is clear. Remove the chicken from the frying pan, let it sit for 5 minutes to cool, and then slice it. This step can be completed one day in advance.

Step 3

When cooking the chicken, stir all the ingredients together in a small bowl or glass jar to make a seasoning. Divide spinach or romaine lettuce into 4 plates (or containers). Recooking preparations, equal parts of black chicken, boiled eggs, tomatoes, cucumbers, mushrooms, red onions, avocado, bacon and blue cheese on top of the greens.

Step 4

Before you serve, serve the salad with 2 tablespoons of red wine vinegar or your favourite condiment.

Per serving: 430 calories, 23 g fat, 45 g protein, 14 g carb, 5 g sugars, 7 g fiber

Spinach Garlic Parmesan Orzo with Crispy Bacon

Ingredients:

- 10 oz. uncooked orzo pasta (about 1 2/3 c. uncooked orzo)
- 8 slices bacon
- ½ c. reserved pasta water, after pasta is done boiling
- 1 tablespoon butter
- ½ c. shredded carrots (or carrots cut into matchsticks)
- 3 cloves garlic, finely minced
- ⅔ c. frozen or fresh sweet corn
- 1 red bell pepper, cut into chunks
- ½ c. freshly grated parmesan cheese
- ½ teaspoon garlic powder
- 1 (5-oz) package organic spinach
- Freshly ground salt and pepper
- ½ teaspoon red chili pepper flakes, plus more if desired

123

Directions:

Step 1

Put the bacon in a large frying pan or pan, place it on medium heat, and cook the bacon on both sides until crispy and brown. If the pot starts to smoke at any time, just lower the heat. After the bacon is cooked, use a paper towel to absorb the excess oil, then cut into small pieces, chopped and set aside

Step 2

When the bacon is cooking, place a pot on high heat and boil on the water, add salt, stir in the pot and cook until all teeth darken for about 10 minutes after the Orzo is cooked, drain the pasta and place it in a colander make sure to reserve a cup of pasta water.

Step 3

Add 1 tablespoon of butter to the same pot where the pasta is cooked and heat it over medium heat. After the butter has melted, add chopped carrots, garlic, red sweet pepper, corn and sauté for 3 minutes.

Step 4

Add spinach and cook until the spinach is wilted for about 3 minutes. Put the cooked Orzo biscuits back into the pot and turn down the heat, add the reserved pasta water, parmesan, garlic powder and red chili pepper flakes and stir.

Step 5

Finally, add the bacon crumbles. Season with salt and pepper. I like to add a lot of black pepper to this dish, it tastes very good. If you think it needs some extra Parmesan cheese, please stir as you please. Enjoy your meal.

Per serving: 363 calories, 14 g fat (6.2 g sat), 20 g protein, 52.7 g carb, 2.6 g sugars,
2.5 g fiber

Instant Pot Beef and Barley Stew

Ingredients:

- 1 tablespoon all-purpose flour
- 1 tablespoon olive oil
- ½ medium butternut squash (1 pound), peeled
- 1 lb. beef chuck, well-trimmed, cut into
- 2-inch pieces
- 1 large onion, chopped
- 4 cloves garlic, smashed
- 8 sprigs thyme, plus leaves for serving
- Kosher salt and pepper
- 3 medium carrots (about 12 ounces), sliced
- 1 12-oz bottle beer and seeded, cut into 2-inch pieces

- 3 cup no-salt-added beef broth
- 1 cup pearled barley

Directions:

Step 1

Put the pot to the sauté. In a medium bowl, toss the beef and flour together then add olive oil to the Instant Pot, then cook the beef until browned on all sides and roast for 6 minutes, then transfer the beef to a plate then add garlic, onion, thyme sprigs and 1/2 teaspoon of salt and pepper, and cook, stirring occasionally, until tender for 5 to 6 minutes. Stir properly

Step 2

Pour the beef into the pot with pumpkin, carrots, beef broth and barley. Close the lid and cook on high pressure for 20 minutes. Use the quick release method to release the pressure. If necessary, sprinkle with thyme.

Per serving: 454 calories, 7g fat (2 g sat), 34 g protein, 330 mg sodium, 67 g carb, 14g fiber

Grilled Chicken with Smoky Corn Salad

Ingredients:

- 1 oz. Manchego cheese, finely grated salt and pepper
- 4 6-oz boneless, skinless chicken breast halves
- 2 tablespoons. chopped green olives
- 2 limes, halved
- 4 ears corn, shucked
- 1/4 c. cilantro, chopped
- 1 1/2 teaspoon olive oil
- 1 teaspoon smoked paprika

Directions:

Step 1

Season the boneless and skinless chicken breasts with salt and pepper, then grill them at a medium-high level for 5 to 6 minutes per side, then, cut the lemon on both sides, after you cut the corn into thin slices, and burn for 6 to 8 minutes.

Step 2

Cut the corn out of the corn cob and place it in a bowl containing half juice of 2 limes halves, then chop the green olives, coriander, chopped Manchego cheese and a little salt and pepper.

Step 3

Serve the chicken with corn, the remaining half of the lime, and a mixture of olive oil and smoked paprika.

Per serving: 335 calories, 13 g fat (3.5 g saturated), 31 g protein, 326 mg sodium, 21 g carb, 2 g fiber

Herb-Roasted Chicken and Cherry Tomatoes

Ingredients:

- 3/4 teaspoon salt
- 1 teaspoon plus 1 tablespoon oil
- 3/4 teaspoon pepper
- 1 sprig rosemary
- 2 large bone-in chicken breasts (about 12 oz. each)
- 1 teaspoon fennel seeds (crushed)
- ¼ c. parsley (chopped)
- 1 c. instant polenta
- 1 lb. cherry tomatoes (halved)
- 1 teaspoon red wine vinegar

Directions:

Step 1

Preheat the oven to 430°F. Heat 1 teaspoon of oil to medium size in a large oven-safe frying pan. Season chicken breasts with ½ teaspoon of salt and pepper. Cook, side down, until golden brown and crispy, for 7 minutes, then add cherry tomatoes, rosemary and fennel seeds, drizzle with 1 tablespoon of oil, then season with ¼ teaspoon of salt and pepper, and roast until the chicken is cooked through and the tomatoes begin to decompose for 15 minutes.

Step 2

At the same time, prepare polenta. Toss in rosemary, then transfer the chicken cutting board and let it sit for 5 minutes, pour red wine vinegar into tomatoes, then add coriander and mix well.

Step 3

Remove the bones from the chicken, slice them into thin slices, place them on the polenta, and serve with tomatoes.

Per serving: 445 calories, 15.5 g fat (2 g saturated), 25 g protein, 325 mg sodium, 37 g carb, 3 g fiber

Cookout for One
 Ingredients:

- 1 organic beef hot dog

- 1 cup sliced honeydew melon
- ½ tablespoon sweet relish
- 1/2 cup organic baked beans
- 1 whole-wheat hot dog bun
- tablespoon whole-grain mustard

Directions:

Step 1

Prepare hot dogs and heat roasted beans in a pot. Put the hot dog in a bun, top with mustard and seasoning, add melon and beans on the side.

Per serving: 350 cal

Summer Farrotto

Ingredients:

- 2 tablespoons olive oil, divided
- 1 tablespoon chopped parsley
- 1 boneless, skinless chicken breast (3 oz.)
- 1/4 cup sliced red onion
- 1 tablespoon grated parmesan cheese
- 1 cup diced yellow squash
- 1/2 cup dry Farro

Directions:

Step 1

Put the chicken in a pot and boil it, with a tablespoon of oil season with salt and pepper, and then cut into small cubes.

Step 2

Fry the onion, then use the remaining oil to press it into thin slices. Stir in the farro until oiled. Add 2/3 cup of water, boil, stir, reduce heat, and cover the pot.

Step 3

Cook until tender. Add chicken, coriander and cheese, stir well and serve.

Per serving: 435 cal

Beef and Veggie Salad Bowl

Ingredients:

- 2 cups Mesclun greens
- ½ cup chopped broccoli florets
- 1/4 red bell pepper, chopped
- 2 teaspoons olive oil
- 3 oz. cooked lean beef, cubed
- 2 tablespoon dry red quinoa

- 1 teaspoon red wine vinegar

Directions:

Step 1

Follow the instructions to cook/prepare quinoa.

Step 2

Put beef, broccoli, greens and pepper into a bowl and stir

Step 3

Stir oil and vinegar evenly.

Per serving: 352 cal

Pork with Veggies

Ingredients:

- 2 tablespoon sliced almonds
- 1 cup steamed green beans
- 1 baked sweet potato
- 1 pork tenderloin (4 oz.)

Directions:

Step 1

Season the pork with salt and pepper, sear in an ovenproof skillet that's coated with cooking spray and transfer to a 430°F oven for 20 minutes.

Step 2

Slice and serve with green beans top it with almonds, and a sweet potato.

Per serving: 374 Cal

Baked Chicken with Mushrooms and Sweet Potato

Ingredients:

- 1 cup baby Portobello mushrooms, sliced
- 1 tablespoon olive oil
- 1 tablespoon chives
- ½ skinless chicken breast
- 1 medium sweet potato

Directions:

Step 1

Bake the chicken with mushrooms, chives and oil in the oven at 320°F for 20 minutes.

Step 2

Microwave the sweet potatoes for 8 minutes.

Per serving: 382 cal

South-western Grilled Chicken Salad

Ingredients

- 1/4 c. light ranch dressing
- 1/4 c. mild green salsa
- 2 tablespoons chopped fresh cilantro
- 1 tablespoon chili powder
- 1/4 teaspoon ground cumin
- 1/4 teaspoon garlic powder
- 1/4teaspoon onion powder
- 1/4 teaspoon salt
- 1 lime, quartered
- 1/4 teaspoon ground black pepper
- 1 lb. thin chicken breast slices or chicken tenders
- 1/2 c. corn kernels
- 6 c. shredded romaine lettuce
- 1 can (15 ounces) black beans, rinsed and drained

* 1 medium tomato, chopped
* thinly sliced red onion

Directions

Step 1

Put the seasonings in a small bowl, then mix the ranch seasonings, salsa and coriander until combined, cover and refrigerate.

Step 2

To make a salad, apply olive oil spray on the grill or ridged roasting pan, and then heat to medium heat. Mix chili powder, onion powder, cumin, garlic powder, salt and pepper in a cup. Rub equally on both sides of the chicken.

Step 3

Roast the chicken, turn it once for 4 minutes, or until it no longer turns pink and the juice becomes clear, transfer to a plate, and then squeeze lime on the cooked chicken.

Step 4

In a bowl, mix the lettuce with half of the dressing then divide it into 4 dishes, sprinkle beans, corn, tomatoes and red onions evenly on each serving, and add grilled chicken on top. Serve the remaining seasoning aside.

Per serving: 235 calories, 24 g protein, 29 g carbs (8 g fiber), 7 g fat (0.4 g sat fat), 4 g sugar, 648 mg sodium

Shrimp, Avocado, and Egg Chopped Salad

Ingredients

- 1/4 small red onion, thinly sliced
- 2 tablespoons. fresh
- lime juice
- 1 tablespoon olive oil
- 12 oz. large peeled and deveined shrimp
- Kosher salt and pepper
- 1 c. grape tomatoes, halved
- 8 c. butter lettuce
- 1/2 c. fresh cilantro leaves
- 1/2 avocado, diced
- 2 hard-boiled eggs, cut into pieces

Directions

Step 1

In a large bowl, mix the onion with lime juice and a tablespoon of oil and let stand for 5 minutes.

Step 2

Heat a tablespoon of oil in a medium-high frying pan. Season the shrimp with ¼ teaspoon of salt and pepper and cook until the whole is opaque, cook for 3 minutes on each side.

Step 3

Put the onion in the tomatoes, then mix well with the lettuce and coriander. Divide into bowls and place shrimp, avocado and eggs on top.

per serving: 325 calories, 21 g protein, 24 g carbs (5 g fiber), 7 g fat (0.4 g sat fat), 4 g sugar, 435 mg sodium

Shrimp Pasta with Salad

Ingredients for pasta:

- ½ cup oil-packed sundried tomatoes, drained and pureed
- ½ cup dry rigatoni, cooked
- 3 oz. shrimp, poached
- 2 teaspoon grated Parmesan
- 3 large black olives, sliced
- 1/2 tablespoon pine nuts

Ingredients for salad:

- 1 cup romaine lettuce
- 1/2 cup sliced cucumber
- ½ Tablespoon balsamic vinegar
- ¼ cup chopped tomato

Directions:

Step 1

Put shrimp, sun-dried tomatoes, olives and pine nuts in the pasta then top with Parmesan cheese. Serve with salad.

Per serving: 325 cal

Seared Scallops with Lemon Juice and Sage

Ingredients:

- 2 teaspoon canola oil
- ½ cups cubed roasted
- ½ teaspoon ground sage
- teaspoon lemon juice
- oz sea scallops
- 2 cups kale sautéed in 2 teaspoons olive oil
- Acorn squash

Directions:

Step 1

Heat canola oil in a large non-stick pan then add the scallops and cook without stirring for about 3 minutes, until browned.

Step 2

Pour in the scallops and cook until the sides are hard and opaque, for 2 minutes, drizzle with lemon juice, and sprinkle some sage on top. Serve with pumpkin and kale.

Per serving: 286 cal

Cheesy Veggie Pasta

Ingredients:

- 1/2 cup low-fat ricotta cheese
- ½ cup whole-wheat macaroni
- cup zucchini wedges
- ¾ cup chopped spinach
- teaspoon olive oil
- 1 cup crushed whole, peeled canned tomatoes

Directions:

Step 1

Prepare vegetables over medium heat, then combine with cooked macaroni and cheese.

Per serving: 329 cal

Eggplant Parmesan

Ingredients:

- zucchini
- ¼ teaspoon sea salt
- tablespoon olive oil, plus more for roasting vegetables
- large eggplant
- 3/4 cup quinoa
- 1/4 cup chia seeds
- 1 cup freshly grated Parmesan, divided
- cups fresh spinach
- 1/4 cup fresh basil
- 1 cup low-fat mozzarella
- ¼ cup chopped fresh oregano
- 1/4 teaspoon freshly ground pepper
- 1 jar marinara sauce (24 oz.), no added salt or sugar

Directions:

Step 1

Peel the eggplant and zucchini, cut into thin slices, brush both sides with oil, and place on a baking sheet, sprinkle salt and bake in a 420°F oven until tender for about 14 minutes.

Step 2

Combine mozzarella cheese, half of Parmesan cheese and oregano. Separately mix quinoa, chia, remaining Parmesan cheese, 2 tablespoons of oil, basil and pepper.

Step 3

Place half of the marinade in the baking dish. Layer half of the vegetables, spinach and cheese oregano mixture. Repeat. Mix quinoa on top and bake for 30 minutes.

Per serving: 260 cal, 17 g fat (4g sat), 36 g carbs, 12 g sugar, 510 mg sodium, 7 g fiber, 14g protein.

Eggplant and Zucchini Lasagna

Ingredients:

- ¼ white onion, diced
- garlic cloves, minced

- cups ricotta cheese • Zest of 1/2 lemon
- can (28 oz.) whole tomatoes, drained
- tablespoon olive oil
- 6 basil leaves, chopped, plus more for serving
- 3 parsley sprigs (leaves only), chopped
- 8 oz. fresh part-skim
- small zucchini, thinly sliced
- small eggplant, thinly sliced
- mozzarella, sliced

Directions:

Step 1

In a medium-high cast iron pan, heat oil, garlic and onions for 3 to 5 minutes, then add tomatoes, stir occasionally until thickened for 5 to 10 minutes.

Step 2

Combine ricotta cheese, zest and herbs in a large bowl, season with salt and pepper. Take out half of the sauce, now put a few layers in the pot half of the vegetable's half of the ricotta cheese and mix then repeat for the rest of the cheese sauce.

Step 3

Bake in a 400°F oven and cover for 20 to 30 minutes until tender. Uncover and bake until bubbling, another 5 to 10 minutes.

Per serving: *326 calories, 18 g fat, 14 g carbs, 5 g fiber, 23g protein.*

Sweet green Portobello, Squash, and Wild Rice Bowl with Ginger Miso Dressing

Ingredients in bowl:

- 2 cups cooked wild rice, warm
- 4 cups kale leaves, shredded
- 1 handful basil leaves, torn
- 3 Portobello mushrooms, stemmed, diced, and roasted
- 1 small butternut squash,
- peeled, diced, and roasted
- 1 small red onion, peeled, diced, and roasted
- 1 medium red beet, peeled and dice.

Ingredients (dressing):
- tablespoon tamari or soy sauce
- thumb-sized piece of ginger, peeled and minced
- ½ teaspoon sesame oil

- ½ cup grape seed oil
- 2 tablespoon rice vinegar
- 2 tablespoons sweet white miso paste
- ¼ cup warm water
- 2 tablespoon mirin
- 1 garlic clove, smashed and minced

Directions:

Step 1

In a blender, mix all seasonings except grape seed oil until uniform. Increase the speed to medium while adding grape seed oil. Set aside

Step 2

Combine all the salad ingredients in a large mixing bowl, and sprinkle with your favourite seasonings. Serve immediately.

Per serving: 322 Cal

Crispy Baked Falafel

Ingredients:

- 1/2 medium onion, chopped
- teaspoon coriander
- ½ c. fresh parsley
- garlic cloves, chopped

- 1 teaspoon cumin
- 1/4 teaspoon black pepper
- 1 teaspoon salt
- 1 c. dried chickpeas, soaked in water overnight
- 1/4 c. vegetable oil

Directions:

Step 1

Preheat the oven to 400°F.

After soaking the chickpeas, drain and rinse with water then add the soaked chickpeas, parsley, onion, garlic, spices, pepper and salt to food processing, pulsate several times until you get a consistent rough texture, make 10-12 small falafel balls by hand.

Step 2

Heat vegetable oil on the stove in the middle pot, and then add the falafel balls. I suggest you do it twice.

Step 3

Cook the falafel balls in the oil for 2 minutes on each side, using a spatula
to carefully flip over, once done, add them to a parchment paper-lined baking dish.

Step 4

Once all the falafels are cooked on the pan and added to the baking dish, drizzle the remaining oil from the pan onto the falafels, and bake for 20 minutes or until browned and crisp. Flip halfway with a spatula.

Enjoy with pita, greens, rice, or your favourite pairings.

Per serving: 128 calories, 6.7 g fat (1.2 g sat), 4.1 g protein, 13 g carb, 261 mg sodium,
2.4 g sugars, 3.7 g fiber

Vegan Chorizo Tostadas

Ingredients:

- 2 tablespoon of chili powder ground dried chili powder
- 4 c. shaved Brussels sprouts
- 2 tablespoon of vegetable oil
- 1/2 teaspoon of ground cumin
- 1 teaspoon of garlic powder
- 1 / 4 teaspoon freshly pepper
- Pinch of ground cloves
- 1 / 2 teaspoon apple cider vinegar
- 1/8 teaspoon ground cinnamon

- Mexican crema (use cashew cream)
- ½ teaspoon salt
- 12 corn tostada shells
- 1 avocado sliced
- 1 c. refried beans

Directions:

Step 1

In a skillet over medium heat add the oil and the shaved Brussels sprouts, leave them until they are soft, like 3 minutes add all the species and mix then well then leave everything for 5 more minutes or until the Brussel sprouts begins to brown on the edges, try not to get them burnt when ready, remove from heat and add the vinegar. Mix and set aside.

Step 2

Put the tostadas together, add 2 tablespoons of black beans, and evenly sprinkle them in the tostadas then add 3 or 4 tablespoons of rich vegan sausage, which is Brussels sprouts with Mexican spices.

Step 3

Drizzle thinly sliced avocado and cashews or tofu pancakes.

Slow Cooker Jamaican Chicken Stew

Ingredients:

- 1 teaspoon curry powder
- ¾ teaspoon ground allspice
- ½ teaspoon red pepper flakes
- ½ teaspoon black pepper
- ½ teaspoon dried thyme
- ½ teaspoon salt
- ½ c. 15 ounces' black beans, rinsed and drained
- teaspoon olive oil
- 1 ½ c. 15 ounces diced tomatoes, un-drained
- lb. chicken parts
- ½ c. red wine
- 1 medium onion chopped
- cloves garlic minced

Directions:

Step 1

Mix chicken with curry powder, thyme, spice powder, red pepper flakes, black pepper and salt.

Step 2

Heat oil in a large frying pan then add the onion and garlic and fry until the onion is soft or about 3 minutes. Add the chicken mixture to the frying pan, brown on both sides. Put wine and cook for a few minutes, add tomatoes and black beans and stir properly.

Step 3

Transfer to a crock pot and cook on high for 5 hours, until tender and the meat falls off the bones.

Step 4

Alternatively, you can continue to cook the chicken on the stove for about 25-30 minutes until it is cooked through.

Per serving: 423 calories, 24 g fat (6 g sat), 32 g protein, 13 g carb, 557 mg sodium, 2 g sugars, 4 g fibre

Spicy Korean Beef Noodle Soup

Ingredients:

- c. cooked short rib meat shredded (from rich beef broth recipe)
- 1.7 oz. mung bean noodles (sometimes called cellophane or glass noodles)
- ½ 2 tablespoon Korean red pepper flakes
- Fish sauce or soy sauce for serving
- 1 tablespoon garlic chopped
- tablespoon toasted sesame oil
- c. Rich Beef Broth
- 1 c. water
- c. bok choy chopped
- scallions cut into 2" lengths
- Extra Korean red pepper flakes for serving
- Fresh shitake mushrooms sliced

Directions:

Step 1

Soak the mung bean noodles in hot water for 20-30 minutes.

Step 2

Heat sesame oil, red pepper flakes and garlic in a small pot until fragrant and garlic turn light brown. Mix with minced meat then keep aside.

Step 3

Heat beef broth and water in a large pot, add the bok choy, mushrooms and drained mung bean noodles, cook for about 3-4 minutes until the noodles are soft and cook the bok choy.

Step 4

Add the marinated meat and spring onions to the soup and heat. Divide into bowls serve with extra Korean red pepper flakes, suitable for spicy food lovers. If the beef broth is not salted, put the fish sauce or soy sauce aside and drizzle it.

Per serving: 312 calories, 8 g fat (5 g sat), 22 g protein, 18 g carb, 677 mg sodium, 1 g sugars, 1 g fiber

Mediterranean Shrimp

Ingredients:

- ¾ teaspoon kosher salt, divided
- ½ teaspoon ground
- black pepper, divided
- 2 tablespoon extra-virgin olive oil
- 2 cloves garlic, minced (about 2 teaspoons)
- 1 teaspoon dried oregano

- 1 lb. large shrimp — 40 to 50 per pound peeled, deveined shrimp, tails on or off (fresh or frozen and thawed)
- 1 14.5-oz. can fire roasted diced tomatoes in their juices
- 1 small red onion — chopped
- ¼ teaspoon red pepper flakes
- 1 teaspoon honey
- 2 Tablespoon fresh lemon juice — from about ½ medium lemon
- ½ c. pitted Kalamata olives
- 1 teaspoon red wine vinegar
- 1 14-oz can artichoke hearts — drained and quartered
- ¾ c. crumbled feta cheese
- 2 tablespoon chopped fresh parsley

For serving:
- Rice — whole wheat couscous, crusty bread, pasta (optional)

Directions:

Step 1

Place a rack in the centre of your oven and preheat the oven to 400°F, Pat the shrimp dry, place in a mixing bowl, and sprinkle with ½ teaspoon salt and ¼ teaspoon black pepper. Toss to coat, then set aside.

Step 2

In a large, ovenproof skillet over medium heat, heat the olive oil then add onion and sprinkle with the remaining ¼ teaspoon salt and ¼ teaspoon black pepper, cook, stirring occasionally, until softened, about 5 minutes, reduce the heat as needed so that the onion softens but does not brown, now add the garlic and cook just until fragrant or for about 30 seconds.

Step 3

Add the tomatoes, oregano, and red pepper flakes, reduce the heat to medium-low and let gently simmer for 10 minutes stir in the red wine vinegar and honey then remove from the heat.

Step 4

Scatter the artichokes and olives over the top, then arrange the shrimp on top in a single layer. Sprinkle with the feta, then bake for 10 to 12 minutes, until the tomatoes are bubbling, cheese has browned slightly, and the shrimp are cooked through.

Step 5

Squeeze the lemon juice over the top and sprinkle with parsley. Enjoy hot.

Per serving: 445 calories, 24 g fat (8 g sat), 38 g protein, 17 g carb, 9 g sugars, 3 g fiber

Mexican Stuffed Peppers

Ingredients:

- 2 teaspoons extra virgin olive oil
- 1 teaspoon ground
- chili powder
- 4 large bell peppers
- 1 teaspoon ground cumin
- 1 teaspoon garlic powder
- ½ teaspoon kosher salt
- 1 can fire-roasted diced tomatoes with juices, 14 ounces
- 1 lb. ground chicken or turkey
- 1 ¼ c. shredded cheese (Monterey Jack, pepper jack, cheddar, or similar cheese), divided
- ¼ teaspoon black pepper
- 1 ½ c. cooked brown rice (quinoa or cauliflower rice)

Directions:

Step 1

Preheat your oven to 375°F, lightly coat a 9x13-inch baking dish with non-stick spray. Slice the bell peppers in half from top to bottom, remove the

154

seeds and membranes, then arrange cut side up in the prepared baking dish.

Step 2

Heat the olive oil in a large, non-stick skillet over medium high heat, add the chicken, chili powder, cumin, garlic powder, salt, and pepper. Cook, breaking apart the meat, until the chicken is browned and cooked through for about 4 minutes then drain off any excess liquid, then pour in the can of diced tomatoes and their juices let simmer for 1 minute.

Step 3

Remove the pan from the heat. Stir in the rice and ¾ cup of the shredded cheese. Mound the filling inside of the peppers, then top with the remaining cheese.

Step 4

Pour a bit of water into the pan with the peppers—just enough to barely cover the bottom of the pan. Bake uncovered for 25 to 35 minutes, until the peppers are tender and the cheese is melted.

Top with any of your favourite fixings, and enjoy hot.

Per serving: 438 calories, 20 g fat (8 g sat), 32 g protein, 32 g carb, 8 g sugars, 5 g fiber

Zucchini Pizza Boats

Ingredients:

- ¼ c. shredded mozzarella cheese — or a blend of shredded mozzarella and provolone
- ¼ teaspoon kosher salt
- c. pizza sauce — or similar prepared marinara sauce
- 4 medium zucchini
- 1 teaspoon Italian seasoning
- teaspoon chopped fresh basil, thyme, or other fresh herbs
- ¼ - ½ tsp crushed red pepper flakes — optional
- ¼ c. mini pepperoni — or mini turkey pepperoni or regular-size pepperoni, sliced into quarters
- 2 teaspoons freshly ground Parmesan

Directions:

Step 1

Place a rack in the centre of your oven. Preheat the oven to 375°F, lightly coat a rimmed baking sheet or 9x13-inch baking dish with non-stick spray.

Step 2

Halve each zucchini lengthwise. With a small spoon or melon baller, gently scrape out the centre zucchini flesh and pulp, leaving a border of about 1/3 inch on all sides, arrange the zucchini shells on

156

the baking sheet. Sprinkle the insides of the zucchini with salt, spoon the pizza sauce into each shell, dividing it evenly, you may need a little more or less, depending upon the size of your zucchini, but don't feel like you need to fill it all the way to the very top.

Step 3

Sprinkle the mozzarella over the top, then evenly sprinkle with Italian seasoning and red pepper flakes (if using). Scatter on the pepperoni and any other desired toppings. Last, sprinkle with Parmesan.

Step 4

Bake for 15 to 20 minutes, until the cheese is hot and bubbly and the zucchini is tender. If desired, switch the oven to broil and cook the zucchini for 2 to 3 additional minutes, until the cheese is lightly browned. Remove from the oven and sprinkle with chopped fresh basil. Serve immediately.

Per serving: 100 calories, 6 g fat (3 g sat), 7 g protein, 5 g carb, 4 g sugars, 2 g fiber

Creamy Gluten-Free Tomato Pasta

Ingredients:

- ½ c. diced white onion
- 1 teaspoon minced garlic
- 10 oz. gluten free past
- Fresh basil and cracked pepper
- ¼ teaspoon each kosher salt and black pepper
- ¼ c. paleo mayo
- 8 oz. canned Italian stewed tomatoes
- (drained)
- 3 tablespoons olive oil (divided)
- 1 egg yolk
- ½ tsp crushed red pepper flakes (optional)

Directions:

Step 1

In a small pot, add onion and garlic to 1 tablespoon of olives and sauté until fragrant or for about 2 minutes, after cooking them, put them aside.

Step 2

a large pot, cook gluten-free pasta according to the instructions, drain the water, rinse the pasta, and then put the pasta back into the pot. Keep calories low, mix the remaining 2 tablespoons of olive oil. Mix properly

Step 3

In another bowl, stir together the mayonnaise and egg yolk, add this mixture to the pan with the pasta and spread until creamy.

Per serving: *353 calories, 17.1 g fat (2.7 g sat), 9.2 g protein, 42.2 g carb, 186 mg sodium, 4.8 g sugars, 3.7 g fiber*

Chinese Cauliflower Fried Rice Casserole

Ingredients:

- 5 oz. diced meat (pork or chicken) (optional)
- 1 tablespoon grated ginger
- Sesame oil for the pan
- 1 small shallot, chopped
- ¼ c. gluten free Szechuan sauce or other gluten free sauce of choice
- 2 teaspoon garlic, minced
- 1 lb. stir fry vegetables
- Handful of mung bean sprouts, optional
- 6 eggs (2 in stir fry and 4 on top, soft baked)
- 3 c. cauliflower rice or broccoli rice (about 1 small to medium head of cauliflower)

- 2 tablespoon beef broth (you can skip if your veggies are less starchy. The broth just gives the casserole more flavor)

Directions:

Step 1

Preheat the oven to 370°F. Add 1-2 tablespoons of sesame oil to a large pot, and heat to medium high. If you want to add meat, please add it here then stir fry until browned and cooked (with sesame oil), then remove the meat and set it aside.

Step 2

If you choose vegetarian food, please skip the browning, then directly add the iron shallot, ginger and garlic to the wok/pan, then stir fry until the aroma is strong-about 2 minutes.

Step 3

Next add all the fried vegetables and seasonings. Stir again for 2-3 minutes until it is evenly oiled, mix the cauliflower rice, broth and 2 eggs together. You can add 2 eggs to the whole fried noodles, or add them after stirring. It's all right, stir-fry for another 3-4 minutes to make fried cauliflower rice. All in all, the cooking time should not exceed 10 minutes, then transfer the ingredients from the wok/pan to an 8 x 11 casserole or baking dish.

Step 4

Crack 4 eggs on the top of the casserole and separate them evenly. Cover with foil and place in 350F oven for 15-20 minutes, or until the eggs are set. For runny eggs, remove the casserole from the oven after baking for 12-15 minutes and cut the egg yolk in the middle to form runny eggs, put the casserole in the oven for another 3-5 minutes.

Step 5

Cool before freezing, or eat immediately. Garnish with green onions, coriander, sesame seeds and optional red pepper flakes.

Per serving: 165 calories, 8.8 g fat (2.4 g sat), 11 g protein, 11.8 g carb, 387 mg sodium, 6 g sugars, 2.8 g fibre

Mexican Salad with Chipotle Shrimp

Ingredients:

- 15 oz. can black beans, drained
- whole ripe avocado, peeled and chopped
- lb. raw jumbo shrimp, peeled and cleaned (tail on or off)
- 8 c. chopped kale

- ¼ c. olive oil
- pint   grape or   cherry tomatoes, halved
- ears corn on the cob, shucked
- 7 tablespoons fresh lime juice, divided
- ½ teaspoon salt
- 2-3 whole chipotle peppers in adobo sauce
- tablespoon honey
- cloves garlic
- ¼ c. mayonnaise

Directions:

Step 1

Preheat the grill to medium heat. In a blender jar, add the jalapeno, 4 tablespoons of lemon juice, olive oil, garlic and salt, cover with puree until smooth.

Step 2

In a separate small bowl, combine 3 tablespoons of chipotle puree and 3 tablespoons of lime juice, Mayonnaise and honey mix until smooth, then season, and add salt and pepper as needed. Prepare all vegetables, place a large salad bowl and add kale, then mix it with the seasoning until the coating is good. (I like to massage the seasoning into the kale with my hands.) Then add black beans, tomatoes and avocado.

Step 3

Place the shrimp and corncob on the grill. *If your shrimp are small, they will fall in the grate. Either use a grill basket or place it on foil.

Step 4

Bake the shrimps for 3-5 minutes until they turn pink. Rotate the corn for 8-10 minutes every 2 minutes. After the corn is cooled enough to handle, cut the corn on the cob and add it to the salad. Then mix the shrimp well and serve.

Per serving: 372 calories, 15 g fat (2 g sat), 31 g protein, 31 g carb, 1314 mg sodium, 9 g sugars, 5 g fiber

Chicken Sausage Apple Squash Sheet Pan Dinner

Ingredients:

- large crisp apple
- Salt and pepper
- 1 sweet onion
- 1 tablespoon olive oil
- 4 chicken sausages
- ½ tablespoon ground allspice
- 1 small butternut squash

Directions:

Step 1

Preheat the oven to 425°F. Cut the butternut squash in half, lengthwise, cut off the round sphere part (the end of the seed pod) and save it for future use.

Step 2

Peel the butternut squash and cut into thin slices. Core the apple, cut into thin slices, and peel. Then peel the onion and slice it into thin.

Step 3

Pile butternut squash, apples, and onions on a wide-sided 18x13-inch "half slice" baking pan. Drizzle olive oil on the top, then beat, spread the pumpkin, apple and onion into a layer. Sprinkle with allspice, salt and pepper then bake in the oven for 15 minutes.

Step 4

At the same time, cut the chicken sausage diagonally into ½-inch slices.

Step 5

Flip the vegetables and spread them out. Make space on the grill pan to add sausage. Return the slices to the oven for 10-
15 minutes, until the sausage sizzles. Serve warm

Per serving: 336 calories, 15 g fat (3 g sat), 15 g protein, 38 g carb, 884 mg sodium, 14 g sugars, 5 g fiber

Confetti Quinoa Stuffed Chicken

Ingredients:

- ⅓ c. shaved unsweetened coconut (coconut chips)
- tablespoon coconut oil
- 4 boneless skinless chicken breasts
- ¾ c. quinoa, any color
- ½ c. chicken broth
- ¾ c. diced bell pepper (red and yellow)
- lime, zest and 1 tablespoon juice
- ½ c. diced red onion
- ¼ c. chopped cilantro
- cloves garlic, minced
- teaspoon chili powder
- 1 teaspoon salt
- 1 serrano pepper, seeded and diced
- 1 teaspoon ground cumin

Directions:

Step 1

Preheat the oven to 375°F. Spread parchment paper on the baked paper on the edges. Put coconut oil in a medium pot and heat it over medium heat. When it melts, add the diced green pepper, red onion, garlic and serrano pepper. Fry for 1-2 minutes to soften a little. Then pour the vegetables into the bowl. They should still be bright in
colour

Step 2

Put the quinoa in the empty seasoning pot. Turn the heat to high, then add the broth and ½ teaspoon salt. Cover the pot and bring to a boil. Cook for 15 minutes or until the broth is absorbed and there are vents on the surface of the quinoa. Remove from the heat, and steam the quinoa for another 5 minutes at the same time, cut a seam in each chicken breast along the long side with a boning knife.

Step 3

Cut the centre of the chicken with a knife parallel to the cutting board, keeping the other side connected. You are trying to create a deep pocket on each breast with a ½ inch border around the three connected sides. Cut into uniform shapes to avoid leaving uncut parts that cannot be cooked in the oven. Then sprinkle cumin, chili powder and salt on each side of each breast.

Step 4

After the quinoa is soft, add the fried vegetables, chopped coconut, coriander, lime zest and lime juice and stir, add salt as needed. Load the confetti quinoa into the cavity of each chicken breast. Place the chicken breast on the baking tray like an open envelope and place the quinoa on top.
Bake for 20 minutes. Serve warm.

Per serving: 355 calories, 13 g fat (8 g sat), 30 g protein, 28 g carb, 1051 mg sodium, 2 g sugars, 4 g fiber

One-Pot Chicken Soup with White Beans & Kale

Ingredients:

- 4 cloves garlic, minced
- 1 c. diced white or yellow onion
- Sea salt and black pepper to taste
- 8 c. broth (chicken broth or vegetable broth)
- 1 15-oz can white beans, slightly drained
- 1 tablespoon avocado oil (if using bacon, omit oil)
- 2 c. shredded chicken
- 1 strip uncured bacon, chopped

- 3 c. loosely packed chopped kale (or other sturdy green)

Directions:

Step 1

Heat a large pot or Dutch oven over medium heat. After heating, add bacon (optional) or oil. Heat for 1 minute while continuing to stir, then add the onion to the Fry for 4-5 minutes, stirring occasionally, until the onion becomes translucent and fragrant.

Step 2

Then add garlic and fry for 2 to 3 minutes, taking care not to burn, next, you add the broth, slightly drain the white beans and chicken, and then cook on a low heat. Cook for 10 minutes to mix the flavour, then season with salt and pepper.

Step 3

In the last few minutes of cooking, add the kale, cover and cook until wilted. Leftovers after cooling can be stored in the refrigerator for 34 days, or in the refrigerator for 1 month. Reheat in the microwave or stove until hot.

Per serving: 201 calories, 6.9 g fat (1.6 g sat), 15.8 g protein, 19.5 g carb, 689 mg sodium, 2.3 g sugars, 15.8 g fiber

168

Balsamic-Marinated Portobello Pizzas

Ingredients:

- ¼ c. balsamic vinegar
- tablespoon avocado or olive oil
- medium red bell pepper (cut into bite-size pieces)
- large Portobello mushrooms (stems removed, wiped clean)
- small red onion (thinly sliced wedges or diced)
- healthy pinch sea salt and black pepper (or red pepper flake)
- head garlic (cloves separated and peeled)
- pinch salt and pepper (or red pepper flake)
- Tablespoon fresh herbs (such as rosemary or oregano optional)
- Tablespoon avocado or olive oil
- ¾ c. pizza sauce
- ⅓ c. soft vegan cheese, divided
- ½ c. sun-dried tomatoes (if large, chop into smaller pieces

Directions:

Step 1

Preheat the oven to 400 degrees Fahrenheit (204 degrees Celsius) and line a large baking sheet with parchment paper. Set aside. Put the Portobello mushrooms (stem facing up) in a shallow dish or large ice bag.

Step 2

Add balsamic vinegar, oil, salt and pepper (or red pepper flakes). Use a pastry brush to paint on all surfaces (or shake the bag to paint). Marinate for 5 minutes on one side first, then for 5 minutes on the other side. At the same time, add vegetables and garlic to the baking tray, then sprinkle with oil, salt, pepper and fresh herbs (optional), then bake for 20-25 minutes or until golden brown and fragrant, and then throw it in the middle Ensure even baking. Set aside, but keep the oven at 400 F (204 C).

Step 3

Heat a large frying pan under the fire (you can also use a grill for this step). Pour the mushrooms into the pot, then save all the remaining oil and vinegar sauce, cook for about 4-5 minutes on each side, or until caramelized and softened. If your mushrooms are particularly thick, covering them can help even cook them completely.

Step 4

Brush with pickled marinade when cooking to inject more flavour. After the mushrooms and vegetables are cooked, assemble the pizza. Place the mushrooms on a baking sheet or a baking sheet lined with parchment paper, and add the toppings, first the pizza sauce, then the roasted vegetables and roasted garlic and soft vegetarian cheese. add vegan Parmesan cheese or red pepper flakes (optional).

Step 5

Bake for about 15-20 minutes or until hot. The top of the vegan soft cheese will be slightly golden. Take it out of the oven and enjoy it directly, or garnish with sun-dried tomatoes, fresh basil, balsamic drizzle, red pepper flakes and vegan parmesan cheese (all optional).

Per serving: 201 calories, 24.6 g fat (2.8 g sat), 4.3 g protein, 22.5 g carb, 134 mg sodium, 14.1 g sugars, 4.2 g fiber

Spicy Tuna Poke Bowls

Ingredients:

- tablespoon reduced sodium soy sauce or gluten free tamari
- ½ lb. sushi grade tuna, cut into ½-inch cubes
- teaspoon sesame oil
- ½ teaspoon sriracha

- ¼ c. sliced scallions
- teaspoon sriracha sauce
- 1 c. cooked short grain brown rice or sushi white rice teaspoon black sesame seeds
- 1 c. cucumbers, (from 2 Persian) peeled and diced
- ½-inch cubes
- tablespoon light mayonnaise
- sriracha,   for   serving optional)
- ½ medium hass avocado, (3 ounces) sliced
- reduced sodium soy or gluten-free tamari, for serving (optional)
- scallions, sliced for garnish

Directions:

Step 1

Mix mayonnaise and Sriracha in a small bowl, dilute with a small amount of water to drizzle.

Step 2

In a medium bowl, mix tuna with green onions, soy sauce, sesame oil and Sriracha. When preparing the bowl, mix it gently and set aside, then in 2 bowls, layer the rice ½ and the tuna ½ layer, avocado, cucumber and green onion.

Step 3

Serve drizzle with spicy mayonnaise and sesame seeds. If needed, add extra soy sauce on the side.

Per serving: 397 calories, 14.5 g fat (2 g sat), 32.5 g protein, 33.5 g carb, 864.5 mg sodium, 3 g sugars, 6 g fiber

Asian Chicken Lettuce Wraps

Ingredients:

- tablespoon rice   wine vinegar
- ¼ c. crushed peanuts, for serving
- teaspoon sesame oil
- 1 tablespoon avocado or olive oil
- 1 tablespoon freshly grated ginger
- tablespoon hoisin sauce
- tablespoon low-sodium tamari (or soy sauce)
- 1 medium onion, diced
- 2 cloves garlic, minced
- 1 tablespoon Sriracha
- 1 lb. ground chicken
- ½ c. water chestnuts, drained and sliced
- butter, bibbs or iceberg lettuce (leaves separated), for serving
- sea salt and black pepper, to taste
- 2 green onions, thinly sliced, for serving

Ingredients for the peanut sauce:

- ¼ c. peanut butter
- clove garlic
- teaspoon Sriracha
- tablespoon low sodium tamari (or soy sauce)
- tablespoon maple syrup
- Water

Directions:

Step 1

Stir hoisin sauce, soy sauce, rice vinegar, Sriracha and sesame oil in a small bowl. Set aside

Step 2

Heat oil in a large frying pan over medium high heat. Add onion and cook until soft, for 5 minutes, then add garlic and ginger, stir, and cook until fragrant for 1 minute. Add ground chicken and cook until it is opaque and most of it is cooked.

Step 3

Chop the meat with a wooden spoon. Stir in the soy sauce and cook for another 1 to 2 minutes, until the soy sauce is slightly reduced and the chicken is fully cooked. Turn off the fire and pour water.

Step 4

Season the mixture, season with salt and pepper if necessary, then put the peanut butter in a small bowl and stir well. For thin sauces, add water 1 tablespoon at a time to achieve the desired consistency.

Step 5

Put the chicken mixture together with lettuce leaves and a spoon into the centre of each leaf about ¼ cup. Topped with peanuts sauce

Per serving: *471 calories, 29 g fat, 28 g protein, 28 g carb, 908 mg sodium, 17 g sugars, 3 g fiber*

Chipotle Chicken Tostadas with Pineapple Salsa

Ingredients:

- Freshly ground salt and pepper
- 2 lb. ground chicken
- 1 tablespoon tomato paste
- 6 (8-inch) grain-free tortillas
- 1 tablespoon avocado oil (or olive oil)
- 2 teaspoon chipotle chili powder
- ½ c. shredded purple cabbage
- ¼ c. chopped fresh cilantro leaves
- avocados, mashed
- ¼ c. low-sodium chicken broth

175

Ingredients for the pineapple salsa:

- 1 tablespoon finely chopped fresh cilantro leaves
- 2 tablespoons fresh lime juice (from 1 lime)
- ¼ c. finely diced red onion
- 1 garlic clove, minced
- 1 tablespoon finely diced jalapeño
- 1 teaspoon avocado oil (or olive oil)
- 2 c. small diced fresh pineapple
- Pinch of salt

Directions:

Step 1

Preheat the oven to 350°F, and line a baking sheet with parchment paper.

Put the pineapple salsa in a medium bowl, add the pineapple, onion, jalapeno, lemon juice, garlic, coriander, and avocado.

Step 2

Mix oil and salt together. Refrigerate until ready to eat, (up to 5 days), boil the chicken, in a large frying pan, heat the avocado oil on medium high heat. Add the ground chicken, chipotle chili powder, salt and pepper.

Step 3

For the cooked chicken, use the back of the spoon to chop the meat until brown, about 7 minutes. If necessary, drain the excess fat from the pan.

Step 4

Reduce the heat to medium, then add chicken broth and tomato sauce and stir well, continue to cook for about 2 minutes or more.

Remove the lid and keep it warm until ready to serve.

Step 5

To Assemble: Place the tortillas in a single layer on the prepared baking sheet. Lightly spray the top of the tortilla with non-stick cooking spray. Bake for 8 to 10 minutes, or until golden brown and crispy.

Step 6

Sprinkle the avocado mashed carefully on each crispy tortilla. Sprinkle with chopped cabbage and a tablespoon of chicken with chestnuts. Top with pineapple salsa and a little cilantro.

Per serving: *462 calories, 26.7 g fat (6.3 g sat), 31.8 g protein,*
26.8 g carb, 7.1 g sugars, 7 g fiber

Creamy Chipotle Sweet Potato Penne Pasta

Ingredients:

- 1/2 tablespoon olive oil
- 1/4 teaspoon garlic powder
- Freshly ground pepper and salt to taste
- c. sliced baby Bella mushrooms
- 1 c. brown rice and quinoa penne

Ingredients for the sauce:

- small roasted sweet potato, skin removed
- ⅔ c. water
- cloves garlic
- ½ teaspoon salt, plus more to taste
- ⅛ teaspoon nutmeg
- ½ c. whole cashews, soaked for 2 hours and drained
- 1 Pueblo Lindo Chiles Chipotle
- Pepper (can add one more if you like extra spice)
- Freshly ground pepper

Directions:

Step 1

Soak the cashews in 4 cups of water for at least 2 hours, otherwise you can put them in a large bowl, then add 4 cups of boiling water, and let the cashews soak in hot water for about 45 minutes to speed up the growth process of cashews

Step 2

When you are ready to make the pasta sauce, add the drained cashews, roasted sweet potatoes, water, garlic, jalapenos, nutmeg, salt and pepper to a high-powered blender. Stir until the thick sauce is combined, then add one or two tablespoons of water, Help fusion if necessary. Taste and adjust seasonings as needed. Leave it for a while.

Step 3

Cook the pasta according to the instructions on the package. Drain the pasta, then pour it back into the pot while the pasta is boiling, sauté the mushrooms, add olive oil to the pan and heat it over medium heat.

Step 4

Add the mushrooms and season with garlic powder, salt and pepper; sauté for 3-5 minutes until the mushrooms are cooked and look juicy.

Stir sweet potato sauce into the cooked pasta. Add mushrooms and stir again, garnish with sage or parsley, whichever one you prefer. Serves.

Per serving: 456 calories, 12.2 g fat (1.8 g sat), 11.4 g protein, 76.9 g carb, 2.8 g sugars, 4.9 g fiber

Spinach Garlic Parmesan Orzo with Crispy Bacon

Ingredients:

- 8 slices bacon
- tablespoon butter
- 10 oz. uncooked orzo pasta (about 1 2/3 c. uncooked orzo)
- cloves garlic, finely minced
- ⅔ c. frozen or fresh sweet corn
- ½ c. reserved pasta water, after pasta is done boiling
- 1 red bell pepper, cut into chunks
- ½ c. shredded carrots (or carrots cut into matchsticks)
- ½ c. freshly grated parmesan cheese
- ½ teaspoon garlic powder
- ½ teaspoon red chili pepper flakes, plus more if desired
- 1 (5-oz) package organic spinach
- Freshly ground salt and pepper

Directions:

Step 1

Put the bacon in a large frying pan or saucepan, heat it over medium heat, and cook the bacon on both sides until crispy and golden brown. If the pot starts to smoke at any time, just lower the heat (or you cook on medium heat). After the bacon is cooked, use a paper towel to absorb the excess oil, then cut into small pieces, cut into small pieces and set aside

Step 2

When the bacon is cooking, place a pot on high heat and add an appropriate amount of salt. Once the water boils, stir in the pot and cook until about 7 to 9 minutes. After Orzo has finished cooking, drain the pasta and place in a colander. Make sure to reserve a cup of pasta water.

Step 3

Next, add 1 tablespoon of butter to the same pot where the pasta is cooked and place on medium heat. After the butter has melted, add chopped garlic, carrots, corn, and red bell peppers and sauté for 2 minutes then add spinach, cook until spinach is wilted, (or about 2 minutes).

Step 4

Also, add in spinach, cook until the spinach wilts, about 2 minutes then put the cooked Orzo biscuits back into the pot and turn down the heat. Pour in the reserved pasta water,
Parmesan, garlic powder and red pepper powder

Step 5

Finally, add the bacon. Season with salt and pepper. I like to add a lot of black pepper to this dish-it tastes very good! If you think it needs some

extra Parmesan cheese, feel free to stir the cup.
Serves

Per serving: 436 calories, 13.3 g fat (6.2 g sat), 20.2 g
protein,
62.7 g carb, 2.6 g sugars, 4.5 g fiber

Rosemary Citrus One Pan Baked Salmon

Ingredients:

- Pinch of ground pepper
- 2 tablespoons fresh orange juice
- 1/3 cup olive oil
- 2 tablespoons fresh rosemary, plus 1-2 extra
- sprigs to garnish
- ½ teaspoon garlic minced
- 1/4 teaspoon of grated dried orange   peel (divided)
- 1   tablespoon Lemon juice
- Kosher salt or fine sea salt to taste
- 1 bunch thin asparagus (trimmed) (or other vegetable of choice)
- 10–12 ounces' sockeye
- salmon (whole fillet or around 3 fillets)
- Olive oil or melted butter to drizzle
- ¼ teaspoon lemon pepper (optional)
- Additional Salt/pepper to taste after baking
- Thinly sliced Orange

Directions:

Step 1

Preheat the oven to 400°F. Stir together orange juice, lemon, 2 tablespoons of rosemary, ¼ to 1/3 cup of olive oil, a little salt, pepper, ¼ teaspoon of orange zest and garlic. Set aside

Step 2

Next, layer the dish, firstly add the chopped asparagus (or other selected vegetables), then drizzle with olive oil or butter, add a pinch (about ¼ teaspoon) of lemon pepper seasoning, place the salmon (skin side down) between the asparagus spears, drizzle orange rosemary marinade on top of salmon.

Step 3

Thinly sliced oranges on salmon and asparagus then put 2 or 2 fresh rosemary sprigs evenly on the salmon and around the pan. Sprinkle more orange peel, pepper, at 400°F. Bake at the same temperature for 12-15 minutes, or until the salmon is no longer opaque in the middle.

Per serving: 345 calories, 22 g fat (3 g sat), 25 g protein, 10 g carb, 5 g sugars, 3 g fiber

Arroz Con Pollo, Lightened Up

Ingredients:

- 1/2 teaspoon adobo powder, Goya
- 2 teaspoons kosher salt to taste
- tablespoon vinegar
- 8 skinless chicken thighs
- 1/2 garlic powder
- teaspoon olive oil
- teaspoon   Sazon, homemade or Badia Sazon tropical
- 1/2 onion
- 1/4 cup cilantro
- 5 scallions
- cloves garlic
- 2 tablespoon bell pepper
- 1 chicken bouillon cube
- 2 ½ cups enriched long grain white rice
- 2 cups water
- 1 medium vine tomato, diced

Directions:

Step 1

Season the chicken with vinegar, ½ teaspoon of sazon, Adobo and garlic powder, and let rest for 10 minutes.

Heat a large and heavy frying pan to medium, add 2 teaspoons of oil when heating then add the chicken and brown eggs for 5 minutes on each side. Remove and set aside.

Step 2

Put the onion, cilantro, garlic, scallions and pepper into the mini food processor. Add the remaining teaspoon of olive oil to the frying pan and sauté on medium low until the onion mixture becomes soft, about 3 minutes.

Step 3

Add tomatoes and cook for some minute then add rice, mix well and cook for one minute, add water, broth (make sure it dissolves well) and remaining sauce, scrape any brown crumbs from the bottom of the pot, to suit your taste, add more as needed.

Step 4

Put the chicken and Nestle into the rice and boil. Cook over medium-low heat until most of the water has evaporated, then you see the liquid on the top of the rice bubbling, then reduce the heat to low heat and cover. Make sure the lid is well sealed and no steam escapes (if the steam escapes, you can put a piece of tin foil or paper towel between the lid and the pot). Cook for 20 minutes without opening the lid.

Step 5

Turn off the heating, and then put the lid on for another 10 minutes (don't peek), Fluff with a fork and eat!

Per serving: 410 calories, 8 g fat (2 g sat), 33.5 g protein, 47 g carb, 655mg sodium, 0.5 g sugars, 1 g fiber

Healthy Greek Chicken and Farro Salad

Ingredients:

- 1 tablespoon olive oil
- 1/2 small red onion, thinly sliced oz. feta, crumbled
- 12 oz. boneless, skinless chicken breasts, sliced ½ inch thick
- ½ seedless cucumber, cut into ½-inch pieces
- 1 tablespoon lemon juice
- Kosher salt and pepper
- ¼ cup   quick-cooking farro
- 1/4 cup fresh dill, chopped
- 8 oz. grape tomatoes, halved
- oz. baby arugula (about 3 cups)

Directions:

Step 1

Cook faro according to package instructions, then drain the water, transfer to a large bowl, and pour 1 tablespoon of oil, meanwhile, in a bowl, toss the onion with 2 tablespoons of lemon juice and a pinch of salt. Sit down and toss twice.

Step 2

Heat the remaining tablespoon of oil in the large saucepan to medium high. Season with salt and pepper, then cook for 8 to 10 minutes, until golden brown then remove the frying pan from the heat and stir in the remaining 2 tablespoons of lemon juice.

Step 3

Add chicken and other juices as well as dill, tomatoes, cucumbers and onions (and their juices) to the farro, toss. Fold with arugula and feta.

Per serving: 380 calories, 10 g fat (1.5 g sat), 26 g protein, 198 mg sodium, 44 g carb, 4 g sugar (0 g added sugar), 7 g fiber

Coconut-Lime Marinated Shrimp + Voodles

Ingredients:

- 3 limes
- 3/4 cup light coconut milk
- cloves garlic
- 1-inch   piece fresh ginger
- red chile
- teaspoon   low-sodium soy sauce
- scallions, thinly sliced, white and green parts separated
- 1 lb. cooked, peeled, deveined shrimp
- medium zucchini
- 1 large, thick carrot
- 1 ½ cup fresh cilantro
- 1 red pepper, sliced thinly

Directions:

Step 1

Cut a lime zest into fines, pour it into a large bowl, and then squeeze all the lime juice (it should produce about ¼ cup), mix in coconut milk and soy sauce then grate in garlic, ginger and ½ red pepper.

Step 2

Chop ½ cup of coriander and pour it into a bowl with the white onion, cut the remaining peppers into thin slices and set aside.

188

Step 3

Use the spiralizer with the thinnest noodle blade to spiral the carrot, and then use the larger blade to spiral the zucchini. Toss the noodles in the coconut milk mixture, let stand for 10 minutes.

Step 4

After 2 minutes, put it in the red pepper, shrimp and remaining coriander. Sprinkle with remaining green onions and thinly sliced peppers.

Per serving: 225 calories, 5.5 g fat (2.5 g sat), 32 g protein, 415 mg sodium, 14 g carb, 7 g sugars, 3 g fiber

Grilled Watermelon + Steak Salad

Ingredients:

- 3 tablespoons fresh lemon
- teaspoon honey
- lb. sirloin (about 1 inch thick)
- 1 lb. cherry tomatoes, halved
- ½ small red onion, thinly sliced
- Kosher salt and pepper
- tablespoon olive oil
- 1 c. fresh mint, leaves torn
- 1/2 small seedless watermelon

- 1 small bunch arugula, thick stems discarded
- 1 c. fresh flat-leaf parsley leaves

Directions:

Step 1

Heat the grill to medium high. Season the steak with ½ teaspoon of salt and pepper per salt, and grill until desired cooked (medium thinning for six to eight minutes per side).

Step 2

Transfer to a cutting board, let stand and cut into thin slices, at the same time, stir lemon juice, oil, honey in a bowl, and then pinch salt and pepper. Cut the onion and tomatoes into thin slices.

Step 3

Cut the watermelon into ½ inch thick triangles, and cut off the peel. Brush lightly with oil, then grill until lightly charred, do that per side. Divide into 4 plates.

Step 4

Fold the herbs into a tomato mixture, then mix gently with arugula. Place the spoon on the watermelon and serve with steak.

Per serving: *361 calories, 18 g fat (4.5 g sat), 28 g protein, 346 mg sodium, 24 g carb, 16 g sugar, 4.5 g fiber*

White Bean and Tuna Salad with Basil Vinaigrette

Ingredients:

- small shallot, chopped
- c. lightly packed basil leaves
- 4 soft-boiled eggs, halved
- 1 tablespoon olive oil
- 12 oz. green beans, trimmed and halved
- Kosher salt and pepper
- 1 tablespoon. red wine vinegar
- 5-oz cans solid white tuna in water, drained
- c. torn lettuce
- 15-oz can small white beans, rinsed

Directions:

Step 1

Bring a large pot of water to a boil. Add 1 tablespoon of salt, then add green beans and cook for 3 to 4 minutes, until soft. Drain the water and rinse with cold water to cool.

191

Step 2

Add lettuce, white beans and tuna, and serve with the remaining seasonings and eggs.

Per serving: 340 calories, 16.5 g fat (3 g saturated), 31 g protein, 770 mg sodium, 24 g carb, 8 g fiber

Rhubarb and Citrus Salad with Black Pepper Vinaigrette

Ingredients:

- tablespoons. honey
- 2 tablespoons. white wine vinegar
- 1/4 c. olive oil
- Kosher salt and pepper
- oz. ricotta salata, shaved
- oz. baby spinach (about 4 c.)
- stalks rhubarb, trimmed
- 1/4 c. toasted pistachios, chopped
- 2 Cara Cara oranges
- 2 bunches watercress, thick stems removed

Directions:

Step 1

In a small bowl, mix the honey and vinegar together. Add rhubarb and stir properly let stand for at least 5 to 10 minutes, then add olive oil, ½ teaspoon salt and 2 teaspoons coarse pepper at the same time, cut the peel and white pith from the orange, and then slice into thin slices.

Step 2

Bowl spinach and watercress fold into orange slices and divide into plates. Scoop out the rhubarb, season each with salad, and sprinkle with pistachios and ricotta cheese.

Per serving: *280 calories, 19.5 g fat (3.5 g saturated), 5 g protein,*
380 mg sodium, 25 g carbohydrate, 4 g fiber

Chicago-Style Chicken Dogs

Ingredients:

- jarred pepperoncini peppers, thinly sliced, plus 1 tablespoon brine
- ¼ small sweet onion, thinly sliced
- teaspoon. yellow mustard, plus more for serving

- teaspoon honey
- 1 teaspoon poppy seeds
- fully cooked   chicken sausages
- small   plum tomatoes, sliced into half-moons
- hot dog buns
- 1 small romaine heart, thinly sliced (about 3 cups)
- dill pickle spears

Directions:

Step 1

Heat the grill to medium temperature. In a bowl, mix the pepper brine, honey and mustard well, add poppy seeds, add pepper and onion and mix well to coat.

Step 2

Grill the sausages, turning from time to time, until lightly charred and heated for 10 to 12 minutes. Bake buns if necessary.

Step 3

Put sausages, tomatoes, and kimchi into the bun. Throw poppy seeds and green onions with romaine lettuce and spoon on the sausage. If needed, serve with the remaining lettuce mixture and mustard.

Per serving: 490 calories, 16 g fat (3 g saturated), 18 g protein, 520 mg sodium, 66 g carb, 6 g fiber

Steak and Rye Panzanella

Ingredients:

- 2 teaspoons. caraway seeds
- 4 tablespoons. olive oil, divided
- tablespoon. wholegrain mustard
- tablespoon. red   wine vinegar
- 1 medium red onion, sliced into rounds
- Kosher salt and pepper
- 1 clove garlic, pressed
- 1 large bunch kale, leaves chopped (about 10 cups)
- 1 bulb fennel, quartered
- slices rye bread (1 inch thick)
- 1 lb. sirloin steak

Directions:

Step 1

Toast the Caraway seeds in a small medium frying pan for about 2 minutes. In a small bowl, mix vinegar, two tablespoons of oil, mustard, garlic, coriander seeds, and teaspoon salt.

Step 2

Heat the grill or grill pan at medium-high temperature. Brush the fennel, onion and bread with 1 tablespoon of oil, then season the fennel and onion with a little salt.

Step 3

Grill, cover the pot, turn it frequently, until the vegetables are tender and burnt and toast the bread. Vegetables need 5 to 8 minutes, and bread needs 1 to 2 minutes. Transfer to a cutting board; peel the fennel, cut into thin slices, and tear the bread into small pieces.

Step 4

In a large bowl, mix the kale, roasted vegetables and bread well, sprinkle half, then set aside and discard from time to time, at the same time, rub the steak with the remaining 1 tablespoon of olive oil and make teaspoons each with salt and pepper. Bake until desired 4 to 6 minutes per side, medium sparsely.

Step 5

Move to a cutting board and let stay for 5 minutes before slicing. Fold into a salad and drizzle with fine vinaigrette

Per serving: 435 calories, 23 g fat (5 g saturated), 29 g protein, 735 mg sodium, 28 g carb, 6 g fiber

Red Curry Shrimp and Cilantro Rice

Ingredients:

- 1 tablespoon. canola oil
- 1 1-inch piece ginger (cut into matchsticks)
- 2 tablespoons. Fresh lime juice
- 1 c. cilantro (chopped)
- 2 cloves garlic (thinly sliced)
- 2 tablespoons. Thai red curry paste
- 1 ½ lb. baby bok choy (4 to 6 heads, trimmed and leaves separated, large leaves halved lengthwise)
- 1 lb. peeled and deveined shrimp
- 1 teaspoon. Grated lime zest
- 1 13.5-oz can light coconut milk
- 1 tablespoon. fish sauce
- 1 c. long-grain white rice

Directions:

Step 1

Cook long-grain white rice. Chop the fluff with a fork and fold in the chopped lime peel and coriander.

197

Step 2

Heat canola oil in a medium frying pan. Add ginger and garlic, stir fry for 2 minutes, then add Thai red curry paste and let cook for 3 minutes. Add light coconut milk and fish sauce and stir for 2 minutes.

Step 3

Add the baby bok choy, peel and remove the shrimp, cook for 3 to 4 minutes, until the shrimp is completely opaque. Add fresh lime juice. If needed, add coriander, red pepper flakes and lime wedges to the rice.

Per serving: 405 calories, 11 g fat (6.5 g saturated), 24 g protein, 1,570 mg sodium, 51 g carb, 4 g fiber

Grilled Pork with Charred Harissa Broccoli

Ingredients:

- 3 tablespoons. plus 1 teaspoon olive oil
- lemons
- ½ lb. pork tenderloin
- Kosher salt
- Pepper
- Tablespoon Harissa
- 1 large head broccoli (about 1 ¼ lbs.), trimmed and cut into large florets

Directions:

Step 1

Heat the grill on medium high. Cut 1 lemon into thin slices, set aside, and then cut two lemons in half. Brush the pork with 1 teaspoon of oil and season with ½ teaspoon of salt. Roast the pork, turning it from time to time until the instant-reading thermometer for 18 to 20 minutes reaches 140°. Transfer to a cutting board and rest for at least 5 minutes.

Step 2

At the same time, coat the broccoli with 1 tablespoon of olive oil and roast with the pork, turning frequently until tender and charred.

Step 3

Grill the lemon until it is charred for 1 to 2 minutes 3. Mix the harissa with the remaining 2 tablespoons of oil, then add the broccoli and mix

Step 4

Cut the lemon in half, then cut pork into thin slices.

Serve with broccoli and roasted lemon cubes.

Per serving: 350 calories, 15.5 g fat (3.5 g saturated), 38 g protein, 375 mg sodium, 8 g carb, 4 g fiber

Bow Ties with Spring Vegetables

Ingredients:

- ¼ cup sliced red
- onion
- 1/2 cup artichoke hearts
- teaspoon olive oil
- 1/4 cup peas
- tablespoon chopped fresh mint
- oz. dry whole-grain farfalle pasta

Directions:

Step 1

Cook the pasta as instructed, and mix with oil, vegetables and mint

Step 2

Add salt and pepper to taste.

Per serving: 360 cal

Half-Homemade Soup with Asparagus

Ingredients:

- 1 cup Amy's Organic Chunky Vegetable soup
- 2 tablespoon dry quinoa

- 1 cup chopped kale
- 10 small asparagus spears
- 2 teaspoon soy sauce
- 1/8 teaspoon grated fresh ginger
- 4 oz. boneless, skinless chicken breast

Directions:

Step 1

Bake the chicken at 350°F for 25 minutes, then chop it with a fork at the same time, put the soup, quinoa and kale in a pot, boil, and then simmer until the quinoa is cooked for about 15 minutes. Add the chicken.

Step 2

Steam the asparagus, then add soy sauce and ginger. Serve the asparagus aside.

Per serving: 340 cal

Light Lasagna

Ingredients:

- 1/2 cup cooked wholewheat spaghetti
- ½ teaspoon crushed red
- chili flakes
- 1/3 cup prepared tomato sauce

- 1 Coleman Natural Mild Italian
- Chicken Sausage link, cooked
- 2 cups spinach
- ¼ cup part-skim ricotta

Directions:

Mix the pasta, ricotta cheese, sauce and paprika together, then chop the sausage. Add spinach for it to wilt.

Per serving: 320 cal

Cilantro Shrimp with Squash, Chard, and Wild Rice

Ingredients:

- Tablespoon olive oil
- teaspoon fresh cilantro
- ¼ cup dry wild rice blend
- 1 yellow squash, sliced
- 8 large shrimp
- 1 cup Swiss chard
- teaspoon fresh lime juice

Directions:

Step 1

Heat the shrimps in olive oil over medium heat for three to four minutes, then season with coriander and lime juice.

Step 2

Steam the pumpkin and chard for five to seven minutes, then cook the rice according to the package instructions.

Per serving: 350 cal

Lemon Chicken with Gazpacho

Ingredients for chicken:

- 3 ½ oz. chicken breast
- 1/2 lemon, sliced
- tablespoon olive oil
- 1 teaspoon fresh rosemary

Gazpacho ingredients:

- 1/2 cup onion, chopped
- 1/4 cup cucumber, chopped
- 1 tablespoon white wine vinegar
- 1/4 cup green pepper, chopped
- 1 cup stewed tomatoes
- 3 cloves garlic, minced

Directions:

Step 1

Coat chicken using olive oil, cover with lemon slices and rosemary, and bake at 350°F for 25 to 30 minutes.

Step 2

Combine gazpacho ingredients in a blender and serve with chicken at room temperature.

Per serving: 306 calories, 7 g fat (6.5 g saturated), 24 g protein, 1,570 mg sodium, 51 g carb, 4 g fiber

Confetti Pesto Pasta

Ingredients:

- 1/3 cup diced chicken breast
- 1/4 cup pesto sauce
- 1/3 cup cooked green beans
- cup cooked linguine
- ¼ pint cherry tomatoes
- ¼ cup shredded Parmesan
- 1/4 teaspoon each salt and pepper

Directions:

Step 1

Put tomatoes, cooked green beans, diced chicken breasts, pesto sauce, salt and pepper into a bowl.

Step 2

Add the cooked linguine and Garnished with shredded parmesan cheese.

Per serving: 206 calories, 7 g fat (6.5 g saturated), 16 g protein, 1,240 mg sodium, 31 g carb, 4 g fiber

Asian Turkey Lettuce Cups

Ingredients for turkey:

- 1/4 cup shelled and cooked edamame
- ½ cup white mushrooms, chopped
- teaspoon minced garlic
- Boston lettuce leaves
- oz. ground lean turkey
- Tablespoon sliced scallion

Ingredients (sauce):

- 1/2 teaspoon rice vinegar
- 1 teaspoon low-sodium soy sauce

- ½ tablespoon hoisin sauce

Slaw Ingredients:

- 1/4 cup grated carrot
- ½ cup shredded red
- ½ teaspoon rice vinegar
- cabbage and green cabbage
- Teaspoon olive oil
- ¼ cup sliced jicama

Directions:

Step 1

In a non-stick pan coated with cooking spray, fry the first three ingredients for 5 minutes.

Step 2

Add edamame, scoop the mixture onto the lettuce, sprinkle with chopped green onion, and wrap. Pour the sauce and place the salad on the side.

Per serving: 239 cal

Mushroom Bison Burger

Ingredients:

- Arnold Artisan Ovens Multi-Grain
- Flatbread
- slices tomato
- 1 portobello mushroom, grilled
- red onion, sliced
- oz. grass-fed bison burger
- lettuce leaves

Directions:

Grill mushrooms and burgers, then sprinkle onions, tomatoes and lettuce on the bread.

Per serving: 254 cal

Salmon with Lemon and Dill

Ingredients:

- ½ cup   chopped
- broccoli, steamed
- 2/3 cup parsnips
- teaspoon dill
- 5 oz wild Atlantic salmon
- 1 tablespoon lemon juice

Directions:

Sprinkle lemon juice and dill on salmon, then bake at 225°F for 15 minutes.

Per serving: 251 cal

Teriyaki Beef with Veggies

Ingredients:

- tablespoon   light honey-mustard dressing
- teaspoon olive oil
- 1/4 cup sliced carrots
- ¼ cup sliced peppers
- oz. grass-fed beef tenderloin, cubed
- 1/2 cup chopped broccoli
- 1/4 cup sliced water chestnuts
- tablespoon reduced-sodium teriyaki sauce
- 1/2 cup cooked brown rice

Directions:

Step 1

Marinate the beef in teriyaki for 30 minutes.

Heat olive oil in a pot and cook the beef for one to two minutes.

Step 2

Add vegetables and cook for another 5 to 7 minutes until the beef is browned. Serve rice.

Per serving: 406 cal

Shrimp and Broccoli Pasta Salad

Ingredients:

- 1/2 steamed broccoli
- ½ teaspoon oregano
- teaspoon capers
- ¼ teaspoon onion powder
- 4 sun-dried tomatoes, halved
- 4 oz cooked shrimp
- tablespoon red wine vinegar
- ½ cup cooked whole-wheat elbow macaroni

Directions:

1. Put all the ingredients in and serve cool.

Per serving: 342 cal

Chicken Parmigiana with Penne

Ingredients:

- 1/2 cup tomato sauce
- ½ cup whole-wheat penne
- 1 cup spinach
- 4 oz. grilled chicken, diced
- 1 ½ tablespoon grated Parmesan

Direction:

Pour spinach into a teaspoon of olive oil, then mix well with chicken, macaroni and tomato sauce. Top with Parmesan.

Per serving: 487 Cal

Jambalaya Blend with Veggies

Ingredients:

- ½ cup chopped red, green, or yellow bell peppers
- Salt to taste
- tablespoon salsa
- ¾ cup diced zucchini

- ½ cup cooked brown rice
- 1/4 cup chopped red onion
- teaspoon olive oil
- tablespoon corn
- ¾ cup diced squash
- veggie burger

Directions:

Step 1

Spray the burger into the pot with cooking spray, then chop the burger and mix it with rice, corn and salsa.

Step 2

Mix the vegetables with oil and salt, roast for 20 minutes, then set aside.

Per serving: 370 cal

Jalapeno Watermelon salad

Ingredients:

- tablespoon balsamic vinegar
- tablespoon extra-virgin olive oil
- c arugula
- tablespoon diced feta cheese
- 1 clove garlic, minced

211

- ½ teaspoon salt
- Watermelon
- c. diced seedless
- ½ c halved cherry tomatoes
- tablespoon apple cider vinegar
- ¼ c. diced red onion
- ¼ teaspoon freshly ground black pepper
- 1 tablespoon seeded and minced jalapeño
- 2 tablespoon minced fresh mint

Directions:

Step 1

Put olive oil, vinegar, garlic, salt and pepper into a large bowl, stir until emulsified

Step 2

Add arugula, watermelon, tomatoes, onions, feta, mint and jalapeno. Toss with your hands can be combined well. Serve immediately.

Per serving: 261 cal, 18 g fat (5 g sat), 14 g carbs, 8g sugar, 440 mg sodium, 1 g fiber, 4g protein.

Spaghetti and Meatballs

Ingredients:

- cup spinach leaves
- cup cooked farro
- 4 egg whites
- 4 tablespoon grated Asiago cheese
- 1 lb. lean ground turkey
- 1 teaspoon oregano
- 4 tablespoon chopped onion
- 1 teaspoon turmeric
- Pinch of salt and pepper
- 4 sweet potatoes

Directions:

Step 1

Preheat the oven to 350°F.

Step 2

To make meatballs, mix the first eight ingredients together by hand, then roll them into 16 balls, each about 1 inch in diameter then place the ball on a pan lined with parchment paper, bake for about 30 minutes or until the top is golden brown.

Step 3

At the same time, wash and peel the sweet potatoes. Then, use a peeler to cut the potatoes into thin ribbons.

Step 4

Put Blanche ribbon in boiling salt water and drain, sprinkle the meatballs on the ribbon and sprinkle them with crushed Asiago. Serve.

Per serving: 327 cal, 5 g fat (1.3 g sat), 34 g carbs, 4 g sugar, 230 mg sodium, 6 g fiber, 35 g protein.

Herb-Roasted Chicken and Cherry Tomatoes

Ingredients:

- ¾ teaspoon salt
- teaspoon, plus 1 tablespoon oil
- ¾ teaspoon. Pepper 1 sprig rosemary
- large bone-in chicken breasts (about 12 oz each)
- 1 teaspoon. Fennel seeds (crushed)
- ¼ c. parsley (chopped)
- 1 c. instant polenta
- 1 lb. cherry tomatoes (halved)
- 1 teaspoon. Red wine vinegar

Directions:

Step 1

Preheat the oven to 430°F. Heat 1 teaspoon of oil to medium size in a large oven-safe frying pan. Season chicken breasts with ½ teaspoon of salt and pepper.

Step 2

Cook, side down, until golden brown and crispy, for 7 minutes, then add cherry tomatoes, rosemary and fennel seeds, drizzle with 1 tablespoon of oil, then season with ¼ teaspoon of salt and pepper, and roast until the chicken is cooked through and the tomatoes begin to decompose for 15 minutes. At the same time, prepare polenta.

Step 3

Throw in the rosemary, then transfer the chicken cutting board and let it sit for 5 minutes, pour red wine vinegar into tomatoes, then add coriander and mix well. Remove the bones from the chicken, slice them into thin slices, place them on the polenta, and serve with tomatoes.

Per serving: 445 calories, 15.5 g fat (2 g saturated), 25 g protein, 325 mg sodium, 37 g carb, 3 g fiber

Cookout for One

Ingredients:

- 1 organic beef hot dog
- 1 cup sliced honeydew melon
- ½ Tablespoon sweet relish

- ½ cup organic baked beans
- 1 whole-wheat hot dog bun
- Tablespoon whole-grain mustard

Directions:

Prepare hot dogs and heat roasted beans in a pot. Put the hot dog in a bun, top with mustard and seasoning, add melon and beans on the side.

Per serving: 350 cal

Summer Farrotto

Ingredients:

- 2 Tablespoon olive oil, divided
- 1 Tablespoon chopped Parsley
- 1 boneless, skinless chicken breast (3 oz)
- ¼ cup sliced red onion
- 1 Tablespoon grated Parmesan cheese
- 1 cup diced yellow squash
- ½ cup dry farro

Directions:

Step 1

Put the chicken in a pot and boil it, with a tablespoon of oil season with salt and pepper, and then cut into small cubes.

Step 2

Fry the onion, then use the remaining oil to press it into thin slices. Stir in the farro until oiled. Add 2/3 cup of water, boil, stir, reduce heat, and cover the pot. Cook until tender. Add chicken, coriander and cheese, stir well and serve.

Per serving: 435 Cal

Beef and Veggie Salad Bowl

Ingredients:

- 2 cups mesclun greens
- ½ cup chopped broccoli florets
- ¼ red bell pepper, chopped
- 2 teaspoons olive oil
- 3 oz cooked lean beef, cubed
- 2 Tablespoon dry red quinoa
- 1 teaspoon wine vinegar

Directions:

Step 1

Follow the instructions to cook/prepare quinoa.

Step 2

Put beef, broccoli, greens and pepper into a bowl and stir

Step 3

Stir oil and vinegar evenly.

Per serving: 352 Cal

Pork with Veggies

Ingredients:

- 2 tablespoon sliced almonds
- 1 cup steamed green beans
- 1 baked sweet potato
- 1 pork tenderloin (4 oz.)

Directions:

Step 1

Season the pork with salt and pepper, sear in an ovenproof skillet that's coated with cooking spray and transfer to a 430°F oven for 20 minutes.

Step 2

Slice and serve with green beans top it with almonds, and a sweet potato.

Per serving: 374 Cal

Baked Chicken with Mushrooms and Sweet Potato

Ingredients:

- 1 cup baby Portobello mushrooms, sliced
- 1 tablespoon olive oil
- 1 Tablespoon chives
- ½ skinless chicken breast
- 1 medium sweet potato

Directions:

Step 1

Bake the chicken with mushrooms, chives and oil in the oven at 320°F for 20 minutes.

Step 2

Microwave the sweet potatoes for 8 minutes.

Per serving: 382 Cal

Southwestern Grilled Chicken Salad

Ingredients

- ¼ c. light ranch dressing
- ¼ c. mild green salsa
- 2 tablespoons chopped fresh cilantro
- 1 tablespoon chili powder
- ¼ teaspoon ground cumin
- ¼ teaspoon garlic powder
- 1/4teaspoon onion powder
- ¼ teaspoon salt
- 1 lime, quartered
- ¼ teaspoon ground black pepper
- 1 lb. thin chicken breast slices or chicken tenders
- ½ c. corn kernels
- 6 c. shredded romaine lettuce
- 1 can (15 ounces) black beans, rinsed and drained • 1 medium tomato, chopped
- Thinly sliced red onion

Directions

Step 1

Put the seasonings in a small bowl, then mix the ranch seasonings, salsa and coriander until combined, cover and refrigerate.

Step 2

To make a salad, apply olive oil spray on the grill or ridged roasting pan, and then heat to medium heat. Mix chili powder, onion powder, cumin, garlic powder, salt and pepper in a cup. Rub equally on both sides of the chicken.

Step 3

Roast the chicken, turn it once for 4 minutes, or until it no longer turns pink and the juice becomes clear, transfer to a plate, and then squeeze lime on the cooked chicken.

Step 4

In a bowl, mix the lettuce with half of the dressing then divide it into 4 dishes, sprinkle beans, corn, tomatoes and red onions evenly on each serving, and add grilled chicken on top. Serve the remaining seasoning aside.

Per serving: 235 calories, 24 g protein, 29 g carbs (8 g fiber), 7 g fat (0.4 g sat fat), 4 g sugar, 648 mg sodium

Shrimp, Avocado, and Egg Chopped Salad

Ingredients

- ¼ small red onion,
- Thinly sliced

- 2 tablespoons fresh Lime juice
- 1 tablespoon olive oil
- 12 oz. large peeled and deveined shrimp
- Kosher salt and pepper
- 1 c. grape tomatoes, halved
- 8 c. butter lettuce
- ½ c. fresh cilantro leaves
- ½ avocado, diced
- 2 hard-boiled eggs, cut into pieces

Directions

Step 1

In a large bowl, mix the onion with lime juice and a tablespoon of oil and let stand for 5 minutes.

Step 2

Heat a tablespoon of oil in a medium-high frying pan. Season the shrimp with ¼ teaspoon of salt and pepper and cook until the whole is opaque, cook for 3 minutes on each side.

Step 3

Put the onion in the tomatoes, then mix well with the lettuce and coriander. Divide into bowls and place shrimp, avocado and eggs on top.

Per serving: 325 calories, 21 g protein, 24 g carbs (5 g fiber), 7 g fat (0.4 g sat fat), 4 g sugar, 435 mg sodium

Shrimp Pasta with Salad

Ingredients for pasta:

- ½ cup oil-packed sundried tomatoes, drained and pureed
- ½ cup dry rigatoni, cooked
- 3 oz shrimp, poached
- 2 teaspoon grated Parmesan
- 3 large black olives, sliced
- ½ tablespoon pine nuts

Ingredients for salad:

- 1 cup romaine lettuce
- ½ cup sliced cucumber
- ½ Tablespoon balsamic vinegar
- ¼ cup chopped tomato

Directions:

Step 1

Put shrimp, sun-dried tomatoes, olives and pine nuts in the pasta then top with Parmesan cheese. Serve with salad.

Per serving: 325 cal

Seared Scallops with Lemon Juice and Sage

Ingredients:

- 2 teaspoon canola oil
- ½ cups cubed roasted
- ½ teaspoon ground sage
- Teaspoon lemon juice
- Oz sea scallops
- 2 cups kale sautéed in 2 teaspoons olive oil
- Acorn squash

Ingredients:

- 1 lb. boneless skinless chicken breasts (3–4 pieces)
- 1 c. grape tomatoes, halved
- 1 large cucumber, sliced
- 1 c. baby Bella mushrooms, sautéed
- ½ c. red onion, chopped
- 1–2 avocados, sliced
- 4 large eggs, hard-boiled, peeled and sliced
- 6 slices cooked turkey bacon, crumbled • ½ c. crumbled blue cheese (optional)

Direction

Step 1

Heat canola oil in a large non-stick pan then add the scallops and cook without stirring for about 3 minutes, until browned.

Step 2

Pour in the scallops and cook until the sides are hard and opaque, 1 minute 2 minutes, drizzle with lemon juice, and sprinkle some sage on top. Serve with pumpkin and kale.

Per serving: 286 Cal

Cheesy Veggie Pasta

Ingredients:

- ½ cup low-fat ricotta cheese
- ½ cup whole-wheat macaroni
- Cup zucchini wedges
- ¾ cup chopped spinach
- Teaspoon olive oil
- 1 cup crushed whole, peeled canned tomatoes

Directions:

Prepare vegetables over medium heat, then combine with cooked macaroni and cheese.

Per serving: 329 Cal

Eggplant Parmesan

Ingredients:

- Zucchini
- ¼ teaspoon sea salt
- tablespoon olive oil, plus more for roasting vegetables
- Large eggplant
- ¾ cup quinoa
- ¼ cup chia seeds
- 1 cup freshly grated Parmesan, divided
- Cups fresh spinach
- ¼ cup fresh basil
- 1 cup low-fat mozzarella
- ¼ cup chopped fresh oregano
- ¼ teaspoon freshly ground pepper
- 1 jar marinara sauce (24 oz), no added salt or sugar

Directions:

Step 1

Peel the eggplant and zucchini, cut into thin slices, brush both sides with oil, and place on a baking sheet, sprinkle salt and bake in a 420°F oven until tender for about 14 minutes.

Step 2

Combine mozzarella cheese, half of Parmesan cheese and oregano. Separately mix quinoa, chia, remaining Parmesan cheese, 2 tablespoons of oil, basil and pepper.

Step 3

Place half of the marinade in the baking dish. Layer half of the vegetables, spinach and cheese oregano mixture. Repeat. Mix quinoa on top and bake for 30 minutes.

Per serving: 260 cal, 17 g fat (4g sat), 36 g carbs, 12 g sugar, 510 mg sodium, 7 g fiber, 14g protein.

Eggplant and Zucchini Lasagna

Ingredients:

- ¼ white onion, diced
- Garlic cloves, minced
- Cups ricotta cheese
- Zest of ½ lemon
- Can (28 oz.) whole tomatoes, drained
- Tablespoon olive oil
- 6 basil leaves, chopped, plus more for serving
- 3 parsley sprigs (leaves only), chopped
- 8 oz fresh part-skim
- Small zucchini, thinly sliced
- Small eggplant, thinly sliced

- Mozzarella, sliced

Directions:

Step 1

In a medium-high cast iron pan, heat oil, garlic and onions for 3 to 5 minutes, then add tomatoes, stir occasionally until thickened for 5 to 10 minutes.

Step 2

Combine ricotta cheese, zest and herbs in a large bowl, season with salt and pepper. Take out half of the sauce, now put a few layers in the pot half of the vegetable's half of the ricotta cheese and mix then repeat for the rest of the cheese sauce.

Step 3

Bake in a 400°F oven and cover for 20 to 30 minutes until tender. Uncover and bake until bubbling, another 5 to 10 minutes.

Per serving: 326 calories, 18 g fat, 14 g carbs, 5 g fiber, 23g protein.

Sweet green Portobello, Squash, and Wild Rice Bowl with Ginger Miso Dressing

Ingredients in bowl:

- cups cooked wild rice, warm
- 4 cups kale leaves, shredded
- 1 handful basil leaves, torn
- 3 Portobello mushrooms, stemmed, diced, and roasted
- 1 small butternut squash, Peeled, diced, and roasted
- 1 small red onion, peeled, diced, and roasted
- 1 medium red beet, peeled and dice.

Ingredients (dressing):

- Tablespoon tamari or soy sauce
- Tablespoon sriracha (optional)
- Thumb-sized piece of ginger, peeled and minced
- ½ teaspoon sesame oil
- ½ cup grape seed oil
- 2 tablespoon rice vinegar
- 2 tablespoons sweet white miso

Paste

- ¼ cup warm water
- 2 tablespoon mirin
- 1 garlic clove, smashed and minced

Directions:

Step 1

In a blender, mix all seasonings except grape seed oil until uniform. Increase the speed to medium while adding grape seed oil. Set aside

Step 2

Combine all the salad ingredients in a large mixing bowl, and sprinkle with your favourite seasonings. Serve immediately.

Per serving: 322 Cal

Crispy Baked Falafel

Ingredients:

- medium   onion chopped
- Teaspoon coriander
- ½ c. fresh parsley
- Garlic cloves chopped
- 1 teaspoon cumin
- ¼ teaspoon black pepper
- 1 teaspoon salt
- 1 c. dried chickpeas, soaked in water overnight
- ¼ c. vegetable oil

Directions:

Step 1

Preheat the oven to 400°F. After soaking the chickpeas, drain and rinse with water then add the soaked chickpeas, parsley, onion, garlic, spices, pepper and salt to food processing, pulsate several times until you get a consistent rough texture, make 10-12 small falafel balls by hand.

Step 2

Heat vegetable oil on the stove in the middle pot, and then add the falafel balls. I suggest you do it twice.

Step 3

Cook the falafel balls in the oil for 2 minutes on each side, using a spatula to carefully flip over, once done, add them to a parchment paper-lined baking dish.

Step 4

Once all the falafels are cooked on the pan and added to the baking dish, drizzle the remaining oil from the pan onto the falafels, and bake for 20 minutes or until browned and crisp. Flip halfway with a spatula.

Enjoy with pita, greens, rice, or your favourite pairings.

Per serving: 128 calories, 6.7 g fat (1.2 g sat), 4.1 g protein, 13 g carb, 261 mg sodium,

Vegan Chorizo Tostadas

Ingredients:

- 2 tablespoon of chili powder ground dried chili powder
- 4 c. shaved Brussels sprouts
- 2 tablespoon of vegetable oil
- 1 / 2 teaspoon of ground cumin
- 1 teaspoon of garlic powder
- 1 /4 teaspoon freshly pepper
- Pinch of ground cloves
- 1 / 2 teaspoon apple cider vinegar
- 1 / 8 teaspoon ground cinnamon
- Mexican crema (use cashew cream)
- 1 / 2 teaspoon salt
- 12 corn tostada shells
- 1 avocado sliced
- 1 c. refried beans

Directions:

Step 1

In a skillet over medium heat add the oil and the shaved Brussels sprouts, leave them until they are soft, like 3 minutes add all the species and mix then well then leave everything for 5 more minutes or until the Brussel sprouts begins to brown on the edges, try not to get them burnt when ready, remove from heat and add the vinegar. Mix and set aside.

Step 2

Put the tostadas together, add 2 tablespoons of black beans, and evenly sprinkle them in the tostadas then add 3 or 4 tablespoons of rich vegan sausage, which is Brussels sprouts with Mexican spices. Drizzle thinly sliced avocado and cashews or tofu pancakes.

Per serving: 268 calories, 11 g fat (4 g sat), 7 g protein, 37 g carb, 314 mg sodium, 3 g sugars, 10 g fiber

Slow Cooker Jamaican Chicken Stew

Ingredients:

- teaspoon curry powder
- ¾ teaspoon ground allspice
- ½ teaspoon red pepper flakes
- ½ teaspoon black pepper
- ½ teaspoon dried thyme
- ½ teaspoon salt
- ½ c. 15 ounces' black beans, rinsed and drained
- Teaspoon olive oil
- 1 ½ c. 15 ounces diced tomatoes, un-drained

- Lb. chicken parts
- ½ c. red wine
- 1 medium onion chopped
- Cloves garlic minced

Directions:

Step 1

Mix chicken with curry powder, thyme, spice powder, red pepper flakes, black pepper and salt.

Step 2

Heat oil in a large frying pan then add the onion and garlic and fry until the onion is soft or about 3 minutes. Add the chicken mixture to the frying pan, brown on both sides. Put wine and cook for a few minutes, add tomatoes and black beans and stir properly.

Step 3

Transfer to a crock pot and cook on high for 5 hours, until tender and the meat falls off the bones. Alternatively, you can continue to cook the chicken on the stove for about 25-30 minutes until it is cooked through.

Per serving: 423 calories, 24 g fat (6 g sat), 32 g protein, 13 g carb, 557 mg sodium, 2 g sugars, 4 g fiber

Spicy Korean Beef Noodle Soup

Ingredients:

- c. cooked short rib meat shredded (from rich beef broth recipe)
- 1.7 oz. mung bean noodles (sometimes called cellophane or glass noodles)
- ½ - 2 tablespoon Korean red pepper flakes
- fish sauce or soy sauce for serving
- 1 tablespoon garlic chopped
- tablespoon toasted sesame oil
- c. rich beef broth
- 1 c. water
- c. bok choy chopped
- scallions cut into 2" lengths
- extra korean red pepper flakes for serving
- fresh shitake mushrooms sliced

Directions:

Step 1

Soak the mung bean noodles in hot water for 20-30 minutes.

Step 2

Heat sesame oil, red pepper flakes and garlic in a small pot until fragrant and garlic turn light brown. Mix with minced meat then keep aside.

Step 3

Heat beef broth and water in a large pot, add the bok choy, mushrooms and drained mung bean noodles, cook for about 3-4 minutes until the noodles are soft and cook the bok choy. Add the marinated meat and spring onions to the soup and heat.

Step 4

Divide into bowls serve with extra Korean red pepper flakes, suitable for spicy food lovers. If the beef broth is not salted, put the fish sauce or soy sauce aside and drizzle it.

Per serving: 314 calories, 8 g fat (5 g sat), 22 g protein, 18 g carb, 677 mg sodium, 1 g sugars, 1 g fiber

Mediterranean Shrimp

Ingredients:

- ¾ teaspoon kosher salt — divided
- ½ teaspoon ground
- Black pepper — divided
- 2 Tablespoon extra-virgin olive oil
- 2 cloves garlic — minced (about 2 teaspoons) •
  1 teaspoon dried oregano

- 1 lb. large shrimp — 40 to 50 per pound peeled, deveined shrimp, tails on or off (fresh or frozen and thawed)
- 1 14.5-oz can fire roasted diced tomatoes in their juices
- 1 small red onion — chopped
- ¼ teaspoon red pepper flakes
- 1 teaspoon honey
- 2 Tablespoon fresh lemon juice — from about ½ medium lemon
- ½ c. pitted Kalamata olives
- teaspoon red wine vinegar
- 1 14-oz can artichoke hearts — drained and quartered
- ¾ c. crumbled feta cheese
- 2 tablespoon chopped fresh parsley

For serving:

- rice — whole wheat couscous, crusty bread, pasta (optional)

Directions:

Step 1

Place a rack in the centre of your oven and preheat the oven to 400°F, Pat the shrimp dry, place in a mixing bowl, and sprinkle with ½ teaspoon salt and ¼ teaspoon black pepper. Toss to coat, then set aside.

Step 2

In a large, ovenproof skillet over medium heat, heat the olive oil then add onion and sprinkle with the remaining ¼ teaspoon salt and ¼ teaspoon black pepper. Cook, stirring occasionally, until softened, about 5 minutes, reduce the heat as needed so that the onion softens but does not brown, now add the garlic and cook just until fragrant or for about 30 seconds.

Step 3

Add the tomatoes, oregano, and red pepper flakes, reduce the heat to medium-low and let gently simmer for 10 minutes stir in the red wine vinegar and honey then remove from the heat.

Step 4

Scatter the artichokes and olives over the top, then arrange the shrimp on top in a single layer. Sprinkle with the feta, then bake for 10 to 12 minutes, until the tomatoes are bubbling, cheese has browned slightly, and the shrimp are cooked through. Squeeze the lemon juice over the top and sprinkle with parsley. Enjoy hot.

Per serving: 445 calories, 24 g fat (8 g sat), 38 g protein, 17 g carb, 9 g sugars, 3 g fiber

Mexican Stuffed Peppers

Ingredients:

- 2 teaspoons extra virgin olive oil
- 1 teaspoon ground
- Chili powder
- 1 large bell peppers
- 2 teaspoon ground cumin
- 1 teaspoon garlic powder
- ½ teaspoon kosher salt
- 1 can fire-roasted diced tomatoes — with juices, 14 ounces
- 1 lb. ground chicken — or turkey
- 1 ¼ c. shredded cheese — Monterey Jack, pepper jack, cheddar, or similar cheese, divided
- ¼ teaspoon black pepper
- 1 ½ c. cooked brown rice — quinoa or cauliflower rice

Directions:

Step 1

Preheat your oven to 375°F, lightly coat a 9x13-inch baking dish with nonstick spray. Slice the bell peppers in half from top to bottom, remove the seeds and membranes, then arrange cut side up in the prepared baking dish.

Step 2

Heat the olive oil in a large, non-stick skillet over medium high heat, add the chicken, chili powder, cumin, garlic powder, salt, and pepper. Cook, breaking apart the meat, until the chicken is browned and cooked through for about 4 minutes then drain off any excess liquid, then pour in the can of diced tomatoes and their juices let simmer for 1 minute.

Step 3

Remove the pan from the heat. Stir in the rice and ¾ cup of the shredded cheese. Mound the filling inside of the peppers, then top with the remaining cheese.

Step 4

Pour a bit of water into the pan with the peppers— just enough to barely cover the bottom of the pan. Bake uncovered for 25 to 35 minutes, until the peppers are tender and the cheese is melted. Top with any of your favourite fixings, and enjoy hot.

Per serving: 438 calories, 20 g fat (8 g sat), 32 g protein, 32 g carb, 8 g sugars, 5 g fiber

Zucchini Pizza Boats

Ingredients:

- ¼ c. shredded mozzarella cheese — or a blend of shredded mozzarella and provolone
- ¼ teaspoon kosher salt
- C. pizza sauce — or similar prepared marinara sauce
- medium zucchini
- 1 teaspoon Italian seasoning
- Teaspoon chopped fresh basil, thyme, or other fresh herbs
- ¼ - ½ tsp crushed red pepper flakes — optional
- ¼ c. mini pepperoni — or mini turkey pepperoni or regular-size pepperoni, sliced into quarters
- teaspoon freshly ground Parmesan

Directions:

Step 1

Place a rack in the centre of your oven. Preheat the oven to 375°F, lightly coat a rimmed baking sheet or 9x13-inch baking dish with non-stick spray.

Step 2

Halve each zucchini lengthwise. With a small spoon or melon baller, gently scrape out the centre zucchini flesh and pulp, leaving a border of about 1/3 inch on all sides, arrange the zucchini shells on the baking sheet.

Step 3

Sprinkle the insides of the zucchini with salt, spoon the pizza sauce into each shell, dividing it evenly, you may need a little more or less, depending upon the size of your zucchini, but don't feel like you need to fill it all the way to the very top.

Step 4

Sprinkle the mozzarella over the top, then evenly sprinkle with Italian seasoning and red pepper flakes (if using). Scatter on the pepperoni and any other desired toppings. Last, sprinkle with Parmesan.

Step 5

Bake for 15 to 20 minutes, until the cheese is hot and bubbly and the zucchini is tender. If desired, switch the oven to broil and cook the zucchini for 2 to 3 additional minutes, until the cheese is lightly browned. Remove from the oven and sprinkle with chopped fresh basil. Serve immediately.

Per serving: 100 calories, 6 g fat (3 g sat), 7 g protein, 5 g carb, 4 g sugars, 2 g fiber

Creamy Gluten-Free Tomato Pasta

Ingredients:

- ½ c. diced white Onion
- 1 teaspoon minced Garlic
- 10 oz gluten free past
- Fresh basil and cracked pepper
- ¼ teaspoon each kosher salt and black pepper
- ¼ c. paleo mayo
- 8 oz canned Italian stewed tomatoes (drained)
- tablespoons olive oil (divided)
- 1 egg yolk
- ½ tsp crushed red pepper flakes (optional)
-

Directions:

Step 1

In a small pot, add onion and garlic to 1 tablespoon of olives and sauté until fragrant or for about 2 minutes, after cooking them, put them aside.

Step 2

In a large pot, cook gluten-free pasta according to the instructions, drain the water, rinse the pasta, and then put the pasta back into the pot. Keep calories low, mix the remaining 2 tablespoons of olive oil. Mix properly

Step 3

In another bowl, stir together the mayonnaise and egg yolk, add this mixture to the pan with the pasta and spread until creamy.

Per serving: 353 calories, 17.1 g fat (2.7 g sat), 9.2 g protein, 42.2 g carb, 186 mg sodium, 4.8 g sugars, 3.7 g fiber

Chinese Cauliflower Fried Rice Casserole

Ingredients:

- 5 oz diced meat (pork or chicken)
- 1 tablespoon grated ginger
- Sesame oil for the pan
- 1 small shallot, chopped
- ¼ c. gluten free Szechuan sauce or other gluten free sauce of choice
- 2 teaspoon garlic, minced
- 1 lb. stir fry vegetables
- Handful of mung bean sprouts, optional
- 6 eggs (2 in stir fry and 4 on top, soft baked)
- 3 c. cauliflower rice or broccoli rice (about 1 small to medium head of Cauliflower)

- 2 tablespoon beef broth (you can skip if your veggies are less starchy. The broth just gives the casserole more flavor.)

Directions:

Step 1

Preheat the oven to 370°F. Add 1-2 tablespoons of sesame oil to a large pot, and heat to medium high. If you want to add meat, please add it here then stir fry until browned and cooked (with sesame oil), then remove the meat and set it aside. If you choose vegetarian food, please skip the browning, then directly add the iron shallot, ginger and garlic to the wok/pan, then stir fry until the aroma is strong-about 2 minutes.

Step 2

Add all the fried vegetables and seasonings. Stir again for 2-3 minutes until it is evenly oiled, mix the cauliflower rice, broth and 2 eggs together. You can add 2 eggs to the whole fried noodles, or add them after stirring. It's all right, stir-fry for another 3-4 minutes to make fried cauliflower rice. All in all, the cooking time should not exceed 10 minutes, then transfer the ingredients from the wok/pan to an 8 x 11 casserole or baking dish.

Step 3

Crack 4 eggs on the top of the casserole and separate them evenly. Cover with foil and place in 350F oven for 15-20 minutes, or until the eggs are set. For runny eggs, remove the casserole from the oven after baking for 12-15 minutes and cut the egg yolk in the middle to form runny eggs, put the casserole in the oven for another 3-5 minutes.

Step 4

Cool down before freezing, or eat immediately. Garnish with green onions, coriander, sesame seeds and optional red pepper flakes.

Per serving: 165 calories, 8.8 g fat (2.4 g sat), 11 g protein, 11.8 g carb, 387.4 mg sodium, 6.2 g sugars, 2.8 g fiber

EAT!

STAY HYDATED!!

EXERCISE!!!

LIVE!!!!